Fat Grafting to the Face for Rejuvenation, Contouring, or Regenerative Surgery

Editor

LEE L.Q. PU

CLINICS IN
PLASTIC SURGERY

www.plasticsurgery.theclinics.com

January 2020 • Volume 47 • Number 1

ELSEVIER

1600 John F. Kennedy Boulevard • Suite 1800 • Philadelphia, Pennsylvania, 19103-2899

http://www.theclinics.com

CLINICS IN PLASTIC SURGERY Volume 47, Number 1
January 2020 ISSN 0094-1298, ISBN-13: 978-0-323-71209-5

Editor: Stacy Eastman
Developmental Editor: Laura Fisher

Clinics in Plastic Surgery (ISSN 0094-1298) is published quarterly by Elsevier Inc., 360 Park Avenue South, New York, NY 10010-1710. Months of issue are January, April, July, and October. Business and Editorial Offices: 1600 John F. Kennedy Blvd., Suite 1800, Philadelphia, PA 19103-2899. Periodicals postage paid at New York, NY and additional mailing offices. Subscription prices are $543.00 per year for US individuals, $987.00 per year for US institutions, $100.00 per year for US students and residents, $607.00 per year for Canadian individuals, $1175.00 per year for Canadian institutions, $655.00 per year for international individuals, $1175.00 per year for international institutions, $100.00 per year for Canadian and $305.00 per year for international students/residents. To receive student/resident rate, orders must be accompanied by name of affiliated institution, date of term, and the *signature* of program/residency coordinator on institution letterhead. Orders will be billed at individual rate until proof of status is received. Foreign air speed delivery is included in all *Clinics* subscription prices. All prices are subject to change without notice. **POSTMASTER:** Send address changes to *Clinics in Plastic Surgery*, Elsevier Health Sciences Division, Subscription Customer Service, 3251 Riverport Lane, Maryland Heights, MO 63043. **Customer Service: 1-800-654-2452 (US and Canada). From outside of the United States and Canada, call 314-447-8871. Fax: 314-447-8029. E-mail: JournalsCustomerService-usa@elsevier.com (for print support); JournalsOnline-Support-usa@elsevier.com (for online support).**

Reprints. For copies of 100 or more of articles in this publication, please contact the Commercial Reprints Department, Elsevier Inc., 360 Park Avenue South, New York, New York 10010-1710. Tel.: +1-212-633-3874; Fax: +1-212-633-3820; E-mail: reprints@elsevier.com.

Clinics in Plastic Surgery is covered in *Current Contents, EMBASE/Excerpta Medica, Science Citation Index, MEDLINE/PubMed (Index Medicus), ASCA,* and *ISI/BIOMED.*

Contributors

EDITOR

LEE L.Q. PU, MD, PhD, FACS
Professor of Plastic Surgery, Division of Plastic Surgery, University of California Davis Medical Center, Sacramento, California, USA

AUTHORS

MAXIME ABELLAN, MD
Plastic Surgery Department, Assistance Publique Hôpitaux de Marseille (AP-HM), Aix-Marseille University, Marseille, France

VALERIA BANDI, MD
Plastic Surgery Unit, Department of Medical Biotechnology and Translational Medicine BIOMETRA, Humanitas Clinical and Research Hospital, Reconstructive and Aesthetic Plastic Surgery School, University of Milan, Rozzano, Milan, Italy

FEDERICO BARBERA, MD
Plastic Surgery Unit, Department of Medical Biotechnology and Translational Medicine BIOMETRA, Humanitas Clinical and Research Hospital, Reconstructive and Aesthetic Plastic Surgery School, University of Milan, Rozzano, Milan, Italy

ANDREA BATTISTINI, MD
Plastic Surgery Unit, Department of Medical Biotechnology and Translational Medicine BIOMETRA, Humanitas Clinical and Research Hospital, Reconstructive and Aesthetic Plastic Surgery School, University of Milan, Rozzano, Milan, Italy

JUNRONG CAI, MD, PhD
Department of Plastic and Cosmetic Surgery, Nanfang Hospital, Southern Medical University, Guangzhou, Guangdong, People's Republic of China

MARCELO CARVAS, MD
Clinique Faria Lima, São Paulo, Brazil

BARBARA CATANIA, MD
Plastic Surgery Unit, Department of Medical Biotechnology and Translational Medicine BIOMETRA, Humanitas Clinical and Research Hospital, Reconstructive and Aesthetic Plastic Surgery School, University of Milan, Rozzano, Milan, Italy

FABIO CAVIGGIOLI, MD
Plastic Surgery Unit, MultiMedica Holding S.p.A., Reconstructive and Aesthetic Plastic Surgery School, University of Milan, Sesto San Giovanni, Milan, Italy

LUIZ CHARLES-DE-SÁ, PhD
ASPS, ISPRES, FILACP, Full Member of the Brazilian Society of Plastic Surgery, Associate Professor of the Department of Plastic, Reconstructive and Aesthetic Surgery, Training and Research State University Hospital of Rio de Janeiro - Brazil (UERJ), Rio de Janeiro, Brazil

MINLIANG CHEN, MD, PhD
Department of Plastic and Burn Surgery, The Third Medical Center of Chinese PLA General Hospital, Beijing, People's Republic of China

CHEN CHENG, MD
Department of Plastic & Reconstructive Surgery, Shanghai Ninth People's Hospital, Shanghai Jiao Tong University School of Medicine, Shanghai, People's Republic of China

STEVEN R. COHEN, MD
Medical Director, FACES+ Plastic Surgery, Skin and Laser Center, La Jolla, California, USA; Clinical Professor, Division of Plastic Surgery, University of California San Diego, San Diego, California, USA

SYDNEY R. COLEMAN, MD, FACS
Department of Plastic Surgery, University of Pittsburgh Medical Center, Pittsburgh, Pennsylvania, USA

RICARDO PICCOLO DAHER, MD, MSc
Division of Outpatient Care, Pronto Socorro para Queimaduras, Goiânia, Goiás, Brazil

SILVIA PICCOLO DAHER, MD
Division of Anesthesiology, Pronto Socorro para Queimaduras, Goiânia, Goiás, Brazil

AURÉLIE DAUMAS, MD, PhD
Internal Medicine Department, Assistance Publique Hôpitaux de Marseille (AP-HM), Aix-Marseille University, Marseille, France

NATALIA DE PAULA PICCOLO, MD
Division of Anesthesiology, Pronto Socorro para Queimaduras, Goiânia, Goiás, Brazil

NELSON DE PAULA PICCOLO, MD
Division of Plastic Surgery, Pronto Socorro para Queimaduras, Goiânia, Goiás, Brazil

PAULO DE PAULA PICCOLO, MD
Division of Plastic Surgery, Pronto Socorro para Queimaduras, Goiânia, Goiás, Brazil

FLORE DELAUNAY, MD
Plastic Surgery Department, Centre Hospitalier du Belvédère, Mont Saint Aignan, France; Aix-Marseille University, Marseille, France

FRANCESCO M. EGRO, MBChB, MSc, MRCS
Department of Plastic Surgery, University of Pittsburgh Medical Center, Pittsburgh, Pennsylvania, USA

ALI GHANEM, MD, PhD
Blizard Institute, Barts and The London School of Medicine and Dentistry, Queen Mary University of London, London, United Kingdom

MICOL GIACCONE, MD
Plastic Surgery Unit, Department of Medical Biotechnology and Translational Medicine BIOMETRA, Humanitas Clinical and Research Hospital, Reconstructive and Aesthetic Plastic Surgery School, University of Milan, Rozzano, Milan, Italy

SILVIA GIANNASI, MD
Plastic Surgery Unit, Department of Medical Biotechnology and Translational Medicine BIOMETRA, Humanitas Clinical and Research Hospital, Reconstructive and Aesthetic Plastic Surgery School, University of Milan, Rozzano, Milan, Italy

NATALE FERREIRA GONTIJO-DE-AMORIM, PhD
ASPS, ISPRES, FILACP, Full Member of the Brazilian Society of Plastic Surgery, Adjunct Professor of Plastic Surgery Course of Pontifical Catholic University of Rio de Janeiro (PUC – Rio) and Carlos Chagas Post-graduation Institute (Pitanguy Institute), Rio de Janeiro, Brazil; Invited Researcher of Verona University - Italy, Verona, Italy

BRIGITTE GRANEL, MD, PhD
Professor, Internal Medicine Department, Assistance Publique Hôpitaux de Marseille (AP-HM), Aix-Marseille University, Marseille, France

XUEFENG HAN, MD, PhD
Plastic Surgery Hospital (Institute), Chinese Academy of Medical Sciences, Peking Union Medical College, Beijing, People's Republic of China

RU-LIN HUANG, MD, PhD
Department of Plastic & Reconstructive Surgery, Shanghai Ninth People's Hospital, Shanghai Jiao Tong University School of Medicine, Shanghai, People's Republic of China

SHU-HUNG HUANG, MD, PhD
Associate Professor, Division of Plastic Surgery, Department of Surgery, Kaohsiung Medical University Hospital, Kaohsiung, Taiwan

SHENGLU JIANG, MD
Department of Plastic and Cosmetic Surgery, Nanfang Hospital, Southern Medical University, Guangzhou, Guangdong, People's Republic of China

SHENGYANG JIN, MD
Plastic Surgery Hospital (Institute), Chinese Academy of Medical Sciences, Peking Union Medical College, Beijing, People's Republic of China

BONG-SUNG KIM, MD
Department of Plastic Surgery and Hand Surgery, University Hospital Zurich, Zurich, Switzerland

FRANCESCO KLINGER, MD
Plastic Surgery Unit, MultiMedica Holding S.p.A., Reconstructive and Aesthetic Plastic Surgery School, University of Milan, Sesto San Giovanni, Milan, Italy

MARCO KLINGER, MD
Plastic Surgery Unit, Department of Medical Biotechnology and Translational Medicine BIOMETRA, Humanitas Clinical and Research Hospital, Reconstructive and Aesthetic Plastic Surgery School, University of Milan, Rozzano, Milan, Italy

YUR-REN KUO, MD, PhD
Professor, Division of Plastic Surgery, Department of Surgery, Kaohsiung Medical University Hospital, Kaohsiung, Taiwan

SU-SHIN LEE, MD
Associate Professor, Division of Plastic Surgery, Department of Surgery, Kaohsiung Medical University Hospital, Kaohsiung, Taiwan

FACHENG LI, MD, PhD
Plastic Surgery Hospital (Institute), Chinese Academy of Medical Sciences, Peking Union Medical College, Beijing, People's Republic of China

MING LI, M. Med
Plastic Surgery Hospital (Institute), Chinese Academy of Medical Sciences, Peking Union Medical College, Beijing, People's Republic of China

QINGFENG LI, MD, PhD
Department of Plastic & Reconstructive Surgery, Shanghai Ninth People's Hospital, Shanghai Jiao Tong University School of Medicine, Shanghai, People's Republic of China

SIN-DAW LIN, MD
Professor, Division of Plastic Surgery, Department of Surgery, Kaohsiung Medical University Hospital, Kaohsiung, Taiwan

TSAI-MING LIN, MD, PhD
Clinical Professor, Charming Institute of Aesthetic and Regenerative Surgery (CIARS), Division of Plastic Surgery, Department of Surgery, Kaohsiung Medical University Hospital, Kaohsiung, Taiwan

YUN-NAN LIN, MD
Division of Plastic Surgery, Department of Surgery, Kaohsiung Medical University Hospital, Division of Plastic Surgery, Department of Surgery, Kaohsiung Municipal Hsiao-Kang Hospital, Kaohsiung, Taiwan

ANDREA LISA, MD
Plastic Surgery Unit, Department of Medical Biotechnology and Translational Medicine BIOMETRA, Humanitas Clinical and Research Hospital, Reconstructive and Aesthetic Plastic Surgery School, University of Milan, Rozzano, Milan, Italy

ROBERTA PICCOLO LOBO, MD
Division of Plastic Surgery, Pronto Socorro para Queimaduras, Goiânia, Goiás, Brazil

FENG LU, MD, PhD
Department of Plastic and Cosmetic Surgery, Nanfang Hospital, Southern Medical University, Guangzhou, Guangdong, People's Republic of China

GUY MAGALON, MD
Professor, Plastic Surgery Department, Assistance Publique Hôpitaux de Marseille (AP-HM), Aix-Marseille University, Marseille, France

JEREMY MAGALON, PharmD, PhD
Culture and Cell Therapy Laboratory, INSERM CBT-1409, Assistance Publique Hôpitaux de Marseille (AP-HM), Aix-Marseille University, Marseille, France

LUCA MAIONE, MD
Plastic Surgery Unit, Department of Medical
Biotechnology and Translational Medicine
BIOMETRA, Humanitas Clinical and Research
Hospital, Reconstructive and Aesthetic Plastic
Surgery School, University of Milan, Rozzano,
Milan, Italy

MASANORI OHASHI, MD, PhD
Chief Surgeon, Aesthetic and Plastic
Department, THE CLINIC Tokyo, Tokyo,
Japan

NORBERT PALLUA, MD, PhD
Aesthetic Elite International – Private Clinic,
Düsseldorf, Germany

CÉCILE PHILANDRIANOS, MD, PhD
Plastic Surgery Department,
Assistance Publique Hôpitaux de Marseille
(AP-HM), Aix-Marseille University, Marseille,
France

MÔNICA SARTO PICCOLO, MD, MSc, PhD
Division of Plastic Surgery, Clinical Director,
Pronto Socorro para Queimaduras, Goiânia,
Goiás, Brazil

NELSON SARTO PICCOLO, MD
Chief, Division of Plastic Surgery, Pronto
Socorro para Queimaduras, Goiânia, Goiás,
Brazil

LEE L.Q. PU, MD, PhD, FACS
Professor of Plastic Surgery, Division of
Plastic Surgery, University of California
Davis Medical Center, Sacramento, California,
USA

YUPING QUAN, MD
Department of Plastic and Cosmetic Surgery,
Nanfang Hospital, Southern Medical
University, Guangzhou, Guangdong, People's
Republic of China

GINO RIGOTTI, MD
ASPS, ISPRES, Chief of Plastic and
Regenerative Surgery, Regenerative Surgery
Unit, San Francesco Clinic, Verona, Italy

J. PETER RUBIN, MD, FACS
Department of Plastic Surgery, University of
Pittsburgh Medical Center, Pittsburgh,
Pennsylvania, USA

FLORENCE SABATIER, PharmD, PhD
Professor, Culture and Cell Therapy
Laboratory, INSERM CBT-1409,
Assistance Publique Hôpitaux de Marseille
(AP-HM), Aix-Marseille University, Marseille,
France

**MARIA THEREZA SARTO PICCOLO, MD,
PhD**
Scientific Director, Pronto Socorro para
Queimaduras, Goiânia, Goiás, Brazil

MATTIA SILIPRANDI, MD
Plastic Surgery Unit, Department of Medical
Biotechnology and Translational Medicine
BIOMETRA, Humanitas Clinical and Research
Hospital, Reconstructive and Aesthetic Plastic
Surgery School, University of Milan, Rozzano,
Milan, Italy

PING SONG, MD
Division of Plastic Surgery, University of
California Medical Center, Sacramento,
California, USA

HIDENOBU TAKAHASHI, MD
Resident, Department of Surgery, Kaohsiung
Medical University Hospital, Kaohsiung,
Taiwan

PATRICK TONNARD, MD, PhD
Director of Coupure Centrum voor Plastische
Chrirugie, Ghent, Belgium

ALESSANDRA VERONESI, MD
Plastic Surgery Unit, Department of
Medical Biotechnology and Translational
Medicine BIOMETRA, Humanitas Clinical
and Research Hospital, Reconstructive
and Aesthetic Plastic Surgery School,
University of Milan, Rozzano, Milan,
Italy

ALEXIS VERPAELE, MD, PhD
Director of Coupure Centrum voor Plastische
Chrirugie, Ghent, Belgium

VALERIANO VINCI, MD
Plastic Surgery Unit, Department of Medical
Biotechnology and Translational Medicine
BIOMETRA, Humanitas Clinical and Research
Hospital, Reconstructive and Aesthetic Plastic
Surgery School, University of Milan, Rozzano,
Milan, Italy

JING WANG, MD
Department of Plastic and Cosmetic Surgery, Nanfang Hospital, Southern Medical University, Guangzhou, Guangdong, People's Republic of China

WENJIN WANG, MD, PhD
Department of Plastic & Reconstructive Surgery, Shanghai Ninth People's Hospital, Shanghai Jiao Tong University School of Medicine, Shanghai, People's Republic of China

HAYLEY WOMACK, DO
MS1 Research Associate, FACES+ Plastic Surgery, Skin and Laser Center, La Jolla, California, USA; Division of Plastic Surgery, University of California San Diego, San Diego, California, USA; Medical Student, Kansas City University of Medicine and Biosciences, Kansas City, Missouri, USA

YUN XIE, MD
Department of Plastic & Reconstructive Surgery, Shanghai Ninth People's Hospital, Shanghai Jiao Tong University School of Medicine, Shanghai, People's Republic of China

SHAOHENG XIONG, MD
Department of Plastic Surgery, Xijing Hospital, Fourth Military Medical University, Xi'an, Shaanxi, People's Republic of China

XIAO XU, MD
Department of Plastic and Burn Surgery, The Third Medical Center of Chinese PLA General Hospital, Beijing, People's Republic of China

ZHIBIN YANG, MD
Plastic Surgery Hospital (Institute), Chinese Academy of Medical Sciences, Peking Union Medical College, Beijing, People's Republic of China

CHENGGANG YI, MD, PhD
Department of Plastic Surgery, Xijing Hospital, Fourth Military Medical University, Xi'an, Shaanxi, People's Republic of China

XINYU ZHANG, MD, PhD
Plastic Surgery Hospital (Institute), Chinese Academy of Medical Sciences, Peking Union Medical College, Beijing, People's Republic of China

LI ZHANQIANG, MD
Director of Mylike Medical Group, Myoung Medical Cosmetic Hospital, Beijing, China

Contents

Facial Fat Grafting: The Past, Present, and Future   1

Francesco M. Egro and Sydney R. Coleman

Fat grafting has evolved over the past two centuries and has revolutionized regenerative medicine, aesthetic and reconstructive surgery. Fat grafting provides a safe and minimally invasive technique to improve signs of aging, sun damage, and congenital and acquired craniofacial deformities. The Coleman technique for harvesting, processing, and grafting provides a reliable strategy for consistent results. However, unanswered questions remain regarding the biology of fat grafting, survival mechanisms, and regenerative properties. The future of fat grafting is bright and includes cell-based therapy and extracellular matrix–based scaffolds. This article provides an overview of the past, present, and future of facial fat grafting.

An Overview of Principles and New Techniques for Facial Fat Grafting   7

Shaoheng Xiong, Chenggang Yi, and Lee L.Q. Pu

Facial fat grafting is a small-volume procedure and is primarily performed for facial rejuvenation, contouring, or regenerative surgery. The unsatisfying retention rate after fat grafting, however, led to unpredictable outcomes, subsequent multiple procedures, and even some complications. A variety of methods have been proposed to enhance the results of facial fat grafting, including several established surgical principles and many possible new techniques. Adding stem cells, fat preparations, and platelet concentrates may improve the survival after fat grafting but randomized controlled clinical studies are needed to determine their safety and efficacy as well as clinical indications for each technique.

Fat Grafting for Facial Rejuvenation: My Preferred Approach   19

Lee L.Q. Pu

The author provides his preferred approach to fat grafting for facial rejuvenation. The preferred donor sites include low abdomen and inner thigh. Fat grafts should be harvested with low negative pressure to ensure the integrity and viability of adipocytes. Fat grafts can be processed with proper centrifugation that can reliably produce purified fat with concentrated growth factors and adipose-derived stem cells, all of which are beneficial to improve graft survival. The approach described in this article is supported by the most scientific studies and thus may provide a more predictable long-lasting result if performed properly.

Fat Grafting for Facial Rejuvenation through Injectable Tissue Replacement and Regeneration: A Differential, Standardized, Anatomic Approach   31

Steven R. Cohen, Hayley Womack, and Ali Ghanem

 Video content accompanies this article at http://www.plasticsurgery.theclinics.com.

Injectable tissue replacement and regeneration (ITR²) is a standardized fat grafting technique, which anatomically addresses losses of facial volume, laxity, and sun damage of the skin resulting from the natural processes of aging. Based on the structural differences of fat existing in the deeper versus the superficial fat compartments of the face, while accounting for skeletal losses and skin aging, ITR^2 utilizes 3 sizes of fat grafts—millifat (parcel size 2.0–2.5 mm), microfat (1.0 mm), and nanofat (<500 μm)—to replicate characteristics of fat cells lost with facial decay and provide increased blood supply and improvements in aging skin.

 Video content accompanies this article at http://www.plasticsurgery.theclinics.com.

Fat grafting is one of the most prevalent fields in facial rejuvenation at present. The procedures include the evaluation of recipient and donor areas, as well as fat harvesting, processing, and reinjection. Inappropriate treatment of each link may affect the final effect on the whole. The authors believe that understanding of facial anatomy and personalized therapy are the key to successful operation.

 Video content accompanies this article at http://www.plasticsurgery.theclinics.com.

Reversing structural changes in aging skin gained potential after the therapeutic use of adipose-derived stem cells was described. Nanofat is a highly concentrated solution of progenitor cells without viable adipocytes. Nanofat grafting creates striking skin quality improvement. The availability of adipose-tissue combined with straightforward mechanical protocol to process fat brings regenerative and antiaging medicine into real-life clinical practice. Association with other cofactors (hyaluronic acid, botulin toxin, and vitamin C) and therapies (microneedling and drug delivery) provides better outcomes. This article describes the techniques and the authors' experiences in nanofat grafting, and its potential new applications in regenerative medicine.

Fat grafting to the face for volume augmentation, and skin rejuvenation have become a popular procedure. However, the main obstacles to fat grafting include the unpredictable volume maintenance rate and the unpredictable number of treatments needed to obtain a satisfactory rejuvenate effect. Therefore, many patients need repeat sessions. However, serial fat grafting with fresh fat imposes a burden on the patient not only because of the pain but also because of the downtime of harvesting. Therefore, if the fat can be cryopreserved, and used many times in 1 harvesting, those burdens can be reduced.

 Video content accompanies this article at http://www.plasticsurgery.theclinics.com.

This study used stromal vascular fraction gel (SVF-gel), a mechanically processed fat-derived product, to treat eye bag and tear trough deformity. SVF-gel is prepared by a process of centrifugation and intersyringe shifting and is particularly rich in SVF cells and native adipose extracellular matrix. SVF-gel injection is used alone or combined with transconjunctival eye bag removal. High satisfaction was noted among patients treated with SVF-gel injection for periorbital rejuvenation with fairly low complication rates. SVF-gel injection is a good alternative to assist transconjunctival lower eyelid blepharoplasty and correct the palpebromalar groove, tear trough deformity, and supraorbital hollow.

 Video content accompanies this article at http://www.plasticsurgery.theclinics.com.

In this article the authors introduce a compartment-based fat graft for facial contouring, focusing on the anatomy of temporal region and midface, the 3L3M integrated fat transfer technique, and the facial compartment-based fat injection in the face. This article includes details of pre-evaluation methods, results of cases, and postoperation care. Readers will have a clear view of how to do facial contouring fat graft in the face after reading this article. There seldom are complications while using the 3L3M technique for fat grafting. The targeted fat grafting can lead to steady and efficient results.

 Video content accompanies this article at http://www.plasticsurgery.theclinics.com.

The concept of microautologous fat transplantation (MAFT), proposed by Lin and colleagues in 2007, emphasized that the volume of each delivered parcel should be less than 0.01 mL to avoid potential fat grafting morbidities. The MAFT-GUN facilitates control of the parcel volume and therefore substantially avoids central necrosis and associated complications. In this article, the authors present a simple, reliable, and consistent procedure based on MAFT for profiloplasty. Favorable outcomes with sustainable long-term effectiveness were obtained, further confirming that the MAFT technique is an alternative for facial contouring in the nose and chin.

Autologous fat graft has limitations, especially long-term unpredictability of volume maintenance. The mechanical enrichment of fat graft with adipose-derived stem cells (ADSCs) could guarantee the survival of fat grafts. After decantation, washing, and centrifugation of lipoaspirate, the authors carried out histochemical analysis and flow cytometry to determine the best layers for preparing ADSC-enriched fat. After centrifugation, the stromal vascular fraction (SVF) was separated by mechanical dissociation and mixed with another layer of intact adipocytes, which was injected into patients. All patients showed volumetric improvement after a single lipotransfer section, without overcorrection. The method is safe, has low cost, and is easily reproducible.

Craniofacial deformities represent a great challenge for the patient and the plastic surgeon. Fat grafting has allowed a shift in paradigm for craniofacial reconstruction by providing a less invasive and safer alternative than traditional reconstructive options. Increasing evidence supports its use with optimal results. This article examines the evidence and practical aspects involved in the decision making and technique of fat grafting to treat secondary craniofacial deformities.

 Video content accompanies this article at http://www.plasticsurgery.theclinics.com.

Reparative, angiogenic, and immunomodulatory properties have been attributed to the cells in the adipose tissue–derived stromal vascular fraction. Because of these characteristics, in the last decade, fat grafting for treatment of autoimmune diseases has grown. This article focuses on systemic sclerosis, a rare autoimmune disease characterized by skin fibrosis and microvascular damage. Lesions of the face are almost always present; however, current therapy is insufficient and patients have considerable disability and social discomfort. This article presents our approach to using fat grafting in the face as an innovative and promising therapy for patients with systemic sclerosis.

Facial fat grafting is increasing worldwide. Although there are few reports in the literature on complications following facial lipofilling, rare but serious complications include embolic risk to local end organs such as the skin and eye, and the central nervous system. Treatment strategies are outlined. The key to prevention of complications is understanding the regional anatomy. It is imperative to adhere to the safe and efficacious techniques to minimize risk. Every surgeon who performs facial fat grafting should establish a systematic method to deliver safe, consistent, and long-term results for their patients.

CLINICS IN PLASTIC SURGERY

ISSUE OF RELATED INTEREST

Facial Plastic Surgery Clinics
https://www.facialplastic.theclinics.com/
Otolaryngologic Clinics
https://www.oto.theclinics.com/

THE CLINICS ARE AVAILABLE ONLINE!
Access your subscription at:
www.theclinics.com

Preface

Fat Grafting to the Face for Rejuvenation, Contouring, or Regenerative Surgery

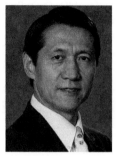

Lee L.Q. Pu, MD, PhD, FACS
Editor

Fat grafting has become one of the most commonly performed procedures in both aesthetic and reconstructive plastic surgery. It started as autologous filler for facial rejuvenation, championed by Dr Sydney Coleman in the mid-1990s, but now it has been used not only for facial rejuvenation but also for facial contouring, another important aspect for facial aesthetic and reconstructive surgery. Until recently, fat grafting has showed its regenerative potential and has also been used to treat some of the difficult clinical problems facing plastic surgeons as an innovative approach called regenerative surgery. As we know more about fat grafting, its mechanisms of how fat grafts survive and their regenerative features, fat grafting, as a relatively noninvasive procedure, may gradually replace many of facial aesthetic and reconstructive procedures in the future. It has become a major armamentarium for plastic surgeons to rejuvenate aged tissues, to contour deficient part of tissues, and to treat certain pathologic conditions of the face.

As a founding member and current board member of International Society of Plastic and Regenerative Surgeons, I believe one of my primary responsibilities is to promote scientific exchange for the art and science of fat grafting. For this reason, I decided to accept another invitation by Elsevier to edit a new issue of *Clinics in Plastic Surgery*. I have chosen the topic of facial fat grafting because this is the most popular anatomic region that fat grafting is frequently performed for rejuvenation, contouring, or

regenerative surgery. I have invited many international contributors who are renowned experts in facial fat grafting not only for facial rejuvenation but also for facial contouring or even for regenerative surgery of the face.

In this issue of 18 articles, the first article, written by Dr Sydney R. Coleman, serves as an introduction on facial fat grafting that includes his perspectives on the past, present, and future of facial fat grafting. This is followed by an article on the overview of current concepts and techniques of facial fat grafting, a good summary of what we know about facial fat grafting, as well as future development in facial fat grafting. There are a total of 6 articles that focus on facial rejuvenation, starting with more established technique and followed by more contemporary and advanced techniques for facial rejuvenation. In addition, facial fat grafting with nanofat grafts, cryopreserved fat grafts, and stromal vascular fraction gel are also included as an individual article. Since facial fat grafting has been commonly used in Asia for facial contouring, a total of 4 articles are included that focus on contouring for temporal region and midface, nose and chin, unilateral face, and even for panfacial contouring. In this issue, an additional 5 articles are included as an innovative approach of regenerative surgery to the face. These articles include fat grafting for treatment of facial burn and burn scars, for treatment of facial scars, for treatment of secondary facial deformity, and last, for treatment of facial scleroderma. The last article focuses on

Clin Plastic Surg 47 (2020) xv–xvi
https://doi.org/10.1016/j.cps.2019.09.003
0094-1298/20/© 2019 Published by Elsevier Inc.

prevention and management of serious complications after facial fat grafting. This article includes unique experiences of our Chinese colleagues, who have been known for the management of serious complications after facial fat grafting. Therefore, this issue represents the most updated information on facial fat grafting for rejuvenation, facial contouring, or regenerative surgery.

As guest editor, I sincerely hope that you will enjoy reading this special issue of *Clinics in Plastic Surgery*. It represents a true team effort from many world-renowned experts from the United States, Greater China, Italy, Belgium, Japan, Italy, Brazil, Germany, and France. I would like to express my heartfelt gratitude to all contributors for their expertise, dedication, and responsibility to produce such a world-class issue of plastic surgery. It is certainly my privilege to work with these respected authors in this exciting field of plastic surgery. I would also like to express my special appreciation to the publication team of Elsevier, who has put this remarkable issue together with the highest possible standard.

Lee L.Q. Pu, MD, PhD, FACS
Division of Plastic Surgery
University of California Davis
2335 Stockton Boulevard, Suite 6008
Sacramento, CA 95817, USA

E-mail address:
llpu@ucdavis.edu

Facial Fat Grafting
The Past, Present, and Future

Francesco M. Egro, MBChB, MSc, MRCS, Sydney R. Coleman, MD*

KEYWORDS

- Facial • Fat grafting • Lipostructure • Lipofilling • Lipoaspirate • Trauma • Reconstruction
- Regenerative

KEY POINTS

- Fat grafting has revolutionized regenerative medicine, aesthetic and reconstructive surgery.
- Fat grafting provides a safe and minimally invasive technique to improve signs of aging, sun damage, and congenital and acquired craniofacial deformities.
- The Coleman technique for harvesting, processing, and grafting provides a reliable strategy for consistent results.
- Many unanswered questions remain in terms of the biology of fat grafting, survival mechanisms, and regenerative properties.
- The future of fat grafting includes cell-based therapy and extracellular matrix–based scaffolds.

THE PAST

The history of facial fat grafting represents a tortuous path in search of a minimally invasive alternative to solve simple and complex soft tissue defects. It is through reflection, criticism, and determination that over the past two centuries fat grafting has gone from being a challenging surgical technique to a beacon of hope for aesthetics, reconstructive surgery, and regenerative medicine.

Fat grafting was first described in 1893 by the German surgeon Gustav Neuber, who transplanted adipose tissue from the arm to the lower orbit to correct unsightly, depressed, and adherent scars caused by osteomyelitis.[1] Although he reported good results, he encountered considerable resorption rates. In 1895, another German surgeon Vincent Czerny described transferring a fist-sized lipoma from the buttock to the breast to improve symmetry following unilateral partial mastectomy for fibrocystic mastitis.[2] In 1910 and 1912, Eugene Holländer reported injections to the face of human fat mixed with ram fat heated to body temperature to correct facial lipoatrophy. He also advocates that should the skin be adherent as occurs in trauma or in bony diseases, the scar between the bone and the skin should be released.[3,4] The German maxillofacial surgeon Erich Lexer used fat and local flaps and cartilage graft to reconstruct the eye socket to accommodate a prosthesis. He subsequently published in 1919 a two-volume book that devoted 300 pages to fat grafting. He described the use of fat grafting for treatment of various pathologies including the treatment facial trauma sequelae, hemifacial microsomia, and treatment of knee ankylosis and tenolysis with fat grafting. This is proof that the reparative and regenerative aspects of fat grafting have been recognized for almost a century.[5] Plastic surgery pioneer Sir Harold Gillies also described in 1920 the use of fat parcels for the reconstruction of

Disclosure Statement: F.M. Egro, nothing to disclose. S.R. Coleman, royalties for instruments sold by Mentor, paid consultant for Mentor Worldwide LLC, and aid consultant for Musculoskeletal Transplant Foundation.
Department of Plastic Surgery, University of Pittsburgh Medical Center, 3550 Terrace Street, 6B Scaife Hall, Pittsburgh, Pennsylvania 15261, USA
* Corresponding author.
E-mail address: sydcoleman@me.com

Clin Plastic Surg 47 (2020) 1–6
https://doi.org/10.1016/j.cps.2019.08.004
0094-1298/20/© 2019 Elsevier Inc. All rights reserved.

various facial wounds with good results.[6] The initial enthusiasm for en-bloc fat transplantation slowed down because of the increasing evidence of fat reabsorption and oil cyst formation, which led to unreliable, hard, and fibrotic tissue. So other facial fillers were attempted through the years including paraffin, silicone, gutta-percha, celluloid, or rubber sponges. Charles C. Miller was one of the first US cosmetic surgeons to use some of these products to correct facial defects, such as crow's feet and nasolabial folds. He also described the use of a piece of adipose tissue harvested from the abdomen and reinjected in facial defects using a special screw piston syringe.[7] However, the use of adipose tissue as injectable did not catch traction until the introduction of liposuction in the 1980s with Pierre Fournier[8] and Yves Gerard Illouz.[9] The adoption of cannulas to remove adipose tissue with a minimally invasive technique was a game changer not only for body contouring but also for the evolution of fat grafting. This allowed reinjection of a more liquid form of fat instead of reinsertion of en-bloc adipose tissue. Despite the innovative harvesting technique, almost complete reabsorption of the fat graft persisted. For this reason, a more systematic approach of harvesting was needed to optimize fat grafting survival, aesthetic outcomes, and minimize donor site morbidity. In 1994, SRC published the technique that would revolutionize the modern aesthetic and reconstructive surgery and open the doors to regenerative medicine.[10]

THE PRESENT

The Coleman technique has been popularized by Coleman since mid-1990s and has been considered, at least by most surgeons, a standardized technique for facial fat grafting. The original technique involved harvesting, purification, and injection with the goal of separating out the unwanted components (oil, blood, local anesthetic, and other noncellular material) through centrifugation and injecting the fat in tiny aliquots with each pass of the cannula. Since its original inception the technique has been refined and improved.

Indications for Facial Fat Grafting

Indications for fat grafting to the face include aging changes, sun damage, and soft tissue deformities. Rhytids are smoothed with intradermal and superficial fat grafting. Orbital and temple hollowing are improved with fat grafting. Volume deficiency (eg, lips) is restored by augmentation. Fat grafting can improve definition of jawline and zygomatic region. Fat grafting can also be used for congenital and acquired soft tissue deformities, such as Parry-Romberg syndrome, craniofacial microsomia, Treacher Collins syndrome, human immunodeficiency virus–related lipodystrophy, scarring, surgical defects, and traumatic soft tissue loss.

Harvesting

Depending on patient preference and the volume of fat required, fat is harvested under either local or general anesthesia. For straight local cases, nerve blocks may be performed. The infiltration solution consists of 0.5% lidocaine with 1:200,000 epinephrine buffered with sodium bicarbonate (or diluted to half the strength to provide a larger volume) infused with a Lamis (or other blunt) infiltration cannula (Mentor Worldwide LLC, Santa Barbara, CA). When intravenous sedation or general anesthesia is required for harvests of larger volumes of fat, the infiltration solution of choice is 0.1% lidocaine with 1:400,000 epinephrine. For either case, the volume of tumescent solution infused should usually be less than the amount of fat to be harvested. A multihole Coleman harvesting cannula attached to a 10-mL syringe is then used to suction the fat. The two-hole cannula originally described in the 1994 paper[10] was replaced by a multihole cannula because of safety concerns because the two-hole cannula would constantly clog and was a safety hazard if dealing with patients with blood infectious diseases. The plunger of the syringe is pulled back only a few milliliters to create enough negative pressure to harvest the fat, while avoiding excessive pressure that could rupture fat cells. On completion of the fat harvest, the incisions are closed with interrupted sutures.

Transfer and Purification

After each 10-mL syringe is filled, the cannula is disconnected, a Luer-Lok cap (Becton, Dickinson and Company, Franklin Lakes, NJ) is placed, and the plunger is removed. Syringes are then placed in a sterilized centrifuge rotor and spun at 1286g for 2 minutes to separate the components of the tissue. The original description of centrifugation at 3400 rpm was replaced by a more accurate gravitational measure because of its increased accuracy (rpm does not take into account the radius of the centrifuge). The centrifugation process concentrates growth factors and stromal vascular fraction (SVF). The oil on the surface is decanted, and the Luer-Lok cap is then removed, allowing the aqueous layer to be drained from the bottom of the syringe. A Codman neuropad (Codman Neuro, Raynham, MA) or Telfa strip (Telfa Strip, Salem, MA) is then placed in the top of the syringe to wick away the remaining oil. The processed fat

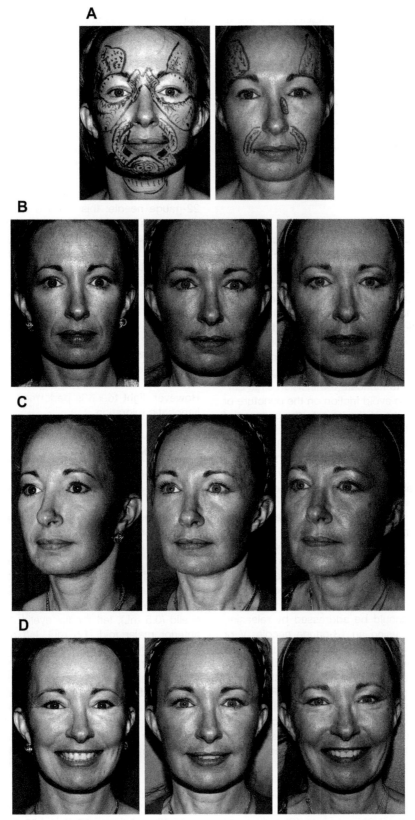

Fig. 1. A 44-year-old woman who has undergone two rounds of facial fat grafting. (*A*) Markings for the initial round (*left*) and second round of fat grafting 2 years later (*right*). The *green marks* demonstrate changes in shape

is then transferred to 1-mL syringes for placement. Centrifugation results in graded densities of the fat, and the highest-density fat remains at the bottom of the 10-mL syringes. Studies have shown better graft take for high-density fat compared with low-density fat.[11] Therefore, when transferring fat from the 10-mL to 1-mL syringes, the injection syringes should be grouped into high-density, intermediate-density, and low-density groups to allow for more thoughtful placement. SRC transitioned from 3-mL to 1-mL syringes because of improved tactile and quantity accuracy in fat delivery.

Infiltration

Incision sites are anesthetized with 0.5% lidocaine with 1:200,000 epinephrine before making stab incisions with a No. 11 blade. A small volume of 0.5% lidocaine with 1:200,000 epinephrine is then infused into graft sites for anesthesia and vasoconstriction. Vasoconstriction reduces the risk of inadvertent intravascular infusion and reduces postoperative bruising. Decanted oil collected during the fat processing stage is used when available to lubricate the incision sites during harvesting to avoid friction on the puncture or incision sites. One of the keys to the success of the Coleman technique is placing the parcels of grafted fat in proximity to an adequate blood supply. To create this environment, fat should be placed in small aliquots surrounded by native tissue. These aliquots should be placed as the microcannula is withdrawn, and no more than 0.1 mL of fat should be placed with each pass. The initial small 17-gauge cannula has been replaced for even smaller ones specifically in facial fat grafting to improve the accuracy of the delivery and because transferring fat parcels that are too large results in fat necrosis, fat resorption, oil cysts, or irregularities. The presence of scar should be addressed by releasing any adhesions using an 18-gauge needle, V or W dissector perpendicularly, and then injecting an appropriate volume of fat into that area. Different depths of fat placement should be used, depending on the desired effect. Fat placed in the intradermal or subdermal layers is ideal to improve wrinkles, and the overall complexion and skin quality. However, at this level, care should be taken to avoid damaging the subdermal plexus and creating superficial irregularities. Fat placed deep against the periosteum is used to change how the remaining soft tissue envelope drapes over the bony structure of the face. Fat placed in the intermediate subcutaneous layers restores volume to rejuvenate or establish a different facial proportion. Molding of the fat placed at any level should be avoided, because this may lead to fat necrosis and resorption. On completion of graft placement, infusion sites are closed with interrupted sutures. A small volume of concentrated fat (approximately 0.2–0.3 mL) is then placed into the closed incisions using a 22-gauge needle; this is done to aid in healing of the incisions. Standard postoperative liposuction garments or compressive dressings are applied to the donor sites to prevent hematoma and seroma formation. For the first 72 hours postoperatively, cool (but not ice-cold) compresses may be applied to the face intermittently to reduce discomfort, bruising, and swelling. Various dressings were initially trialed but most were cumbersome and no benefit was noticed. Thus, facial dressings were abandoned all together. Deep massage of the face should be avoided, because it can cause fat migration or necrosis. However, light touch is performed to encourage lymphatic migration.

Case Demonstration

A 44-year-old woman with a past medical history of face-lift and lower and upper lid blepharoplasty presented with hollowing of the orbits, tear troughs, deepening of her nasolabial folds, loss of malar prominence, perioral rhytids, marionette lines, and loss of definition of her jawline. A total of 200 mL fat was harvested from her thighs and knees and processed using the Coleman technique. Fat was grafted in the right temple (6 mL), left temple (6 mL), glabella (1.5 mL), right medial eyelid (0.5 mL), left medial eyelid (0.5 mL), right anterior malar fold (1.5 mL), left anterior malar fold (1.5 mL), right anterior malar region (3 mL), left anterior malar region (4 mL), right lateral malar region (7 mL), left lateral malar region (8 mL), right nasolabial fold (7 mL), left nasolabial fold (5 mL), right buccal cheek (6 mL), left buccal cheek (4 mL), right mandibular jawline (4 mL), left mandibular jawline (4 mL), mental groove (0.5 mL), and submental region (6 mL). Two years

and size, and the *orange borders* demonstrate the limits of placement. (*B*) Preoperative photographs of the initial round (*left*) and second round of fat grafting 22 months later (*center*), and 10-year follow-up after her second procedure (*right*). (*C*) Oblique views. (*D*) Actively smiling views. (*From* Coleman SR, Katzel EB. Fat grafting for facial filling and regeneration. Clin Plast Surg 2015;42(3):295–6; with permission.)

later the patient was pleased with the result but desired minor enhancements. A total volume of 40 mL was harvested and grafted in the right temple (4.7 mL), left temple (3.5 mL), left side of her nose (0.6 mL), right nasolabial fold (1 mL), and left nasolabial fold (3 mL). Preoperative and 10-year postoperative photographs are shown in **Fig. 1**. The patient has a lasting volume restoration and skin quality improvement.

THE FUTURE

Clinicians and researchers are just scratching the surface of the rejuvenating, reconstructive, and regenerating potential of fat grafting to the face. Fat grafting has proven to be a safe and minimally invasive alternative to complex and open procedures. It provides optimal and long-lasting results for signs of aging, sun damage, and congenital and acquired craniofacial deformities. In the aesthetic realm will be seen a greater role of fat grafting in combination with other procedures, such as facelifts and blepharoplasty, to address signs of aging in the lids, cheeks, tear trough, nasolabial fold, and perioral region that are harder to correct with current surgical techniques. Fat grafting will also be increasingly used to improve the quality of skin. The exact mechanism remains unclear but the senior author has found over the years a significant improvement in quality, texture, and color of the skin as demonstrated in **Fig. 1**. In the reconstructive realm fat grafting has been increasingly used alone or in conjunction with local and distant flaps. Craniofacial surgeons are increasingly using it for reconstruction of congenital deformities, such as Parry-Romberg syndrome or hemifacial microsomia, replacing the need for complex flap reconstruction.[12] Head and neck cancer reconstruction has seen an increase in use of fat grafting to improve the contour of head and neck reconstruction, improve the quality of the skin and soft tissues following radiation, and to prevent hardware extrusion.[13] Traumatic and surgical secondary deformities are increasingly managed with fat grafting to restore form and function with optimal aesthetic results and fat survival.[14]

A variety of strategies have been attempted to improve fat grafting outcomes and survival including the addition of adipose-derived stem cells (ASC), SVF, and platelet-rich plasma. Current evidence is predominantly from animal-based studies rather than from clinical studies, and significant inconsistencies in study methodology exist across human studies, which prevent us from direct comparison and making definitive conclusions.[15] The angiogenic and immunomodulatory influence of ASCs has great potential to improve facial fat grafting outcomes. However, current Food and Drug Administration regulations and additional costs prevent the use of ASC and SVF in the nonresearch setting. Once cost, processing technique, and regulatory barriers are overcome these human cell-based therapies will become increasingly popular and will open avenues to improve fat graft survival, wound healing, and more. An interesting prospect is the development of an off-the-shelf fat grafting product to provide an easy and safe alternative to fat grafting. Over the years, various extracellular matrix–based scaffolds have been commercialized including decellularized adipose tissue scaffold. Recently, our group published animal and human outcomes of a human allograft adipose tissue matrix, demonstrating its adipoinduction potential and optimal volume retention.[16] More studies are needed but the potential of avoiding donor site morbidity associated with fat harvesting is appealing to the surgeon and the patient.

SUMMARY

Fat grafting has significantly evolved over the past century and has proven to have not only anatomic but also functional purpose. The Coleman technique has provided a framework for facial fat grafting allowing standardization and more predictable results. Many unanswered questions remain in terms of the biology of fat grafting, survival mechanisms, and regenerative properties but we look forward to the increasing volume of research to provide these answers. The innovations in adipose tissue and cell-based therapy have opened new doors to regenerative medicine and aesthetic and reconstructive surgery and we foresee a bright future for our specialty.

REFERENCES

1. Neuber GA. Fetttransplantation. Chir Kongr Verhandl Deutsche Gesellschaft für Chirurgie 1893;22:66.
2. Czerny V. Plastischer Erzats de Brustdruse durch ein Lipom. Zentralbl Chir 1895;27:72.
3. Holländer E. Über einen Fall von fortschreitenden Schwund des Fettgewebes und seinen kosmetischen Ersatz durch Menschenfett. Münch Med Wochenschr 1910;57:1794–5.
4. Holländer E. Die kosmetische Chirurgie. In: Joseph M, editor. Handbuch der Kosmetik. Leipzig (Germany): von Veit; 1912. p. 689–90, 708.
5. Lexer E. Die freien transplantationen. Stuttgart (Germany): Enke; 1919–1924.
6. Gillies HD. Plastic surgery of the face. London: Frowde, Hodder, Stoughton; 1920.

7. Miller CC. Cannula implants and review of implantation technics in esthetic surgery. Chicago: Oak Press; 1926. p. 25–30, 66–71.

8. Fournier PF. Microlipoextraction et microlipoinjection. Rev Cir Esthét Langue 1985;10:36–40.

9. Illouz YG. The fat cell "graft": a new technique to fill depressions. Plast Reconstr Surg 1986;78:122–3.

10. Coleman SR. The technique of periorbital lipoinfiltration. Oper Techn Plast Surg 1994;1:120–6.

11. Allen RJ Jr, Canizares O Jr, Scharf C, et al. Grading lipoaspirate: is there an optimal density for fat grafting? Plast Reconstr Surg 2013;131(1):38–45.

12. Denadai R, Raposo-Amaral CA, Raposo-Amaral CE. Fat grafting in managing craniofacial deformities. Plast Reconstr Surg 2019;143(5):1447–55.

13. Karmali RJ, Hanson SE, Nguyen AT, et al. Outcomes following autologous fat grafting for oncologic head and neck reconstruction. Plast Reconstr Surg 2018; 142(3):771–80.

14. Bourne DA, Bliley J, James I, et al. Changing the paradigm of craniofacial reconstruction: a prospective clinical trial of autologous fat transfer for craniofacial deformities. Ann Surg 2019. [Epub ahead of print].

15. Brooker JE, Rubin JP, Marra KG, et al. The future of facial fat grafting. J Craniofac Surg 2019;30(3): 644–51.

16. Kokai LE, Schilling BK, Chnari E, et al. Injectable allograft adipose matrix supports adipogenic tissue remodeling in the nude mouse and human. Plast Reconstr Surg 2019;143(2):299e–309e.

An Overview of Principles and New Techniques for Facial Fat Grafting

Shaoheng Xiong, MD[a], Chenggang Yi, MD, PhD[a],*, Lee L.Q. Pu, MD, PhD[b],*

KEYWORDS

- Facial fat grafting • Surgical principle • Surgical technique • Coleman technique • Nanofat/SVF-gel
- Platelet-rich plasma • Platelet concentrates

KEY POINTS

- Fat grafts should be processed with centrifugation that can reliably produce high-density fat, which concentrates adipose-derived stem cells and reduces inflammatory response, all of which are beneficial to graft retention.
- Stem cells, such as adipose-derived stem cells and bone marrow–derived stem cells, have been reported to be cotransplanted with facial fat grafting, but the efficacy and safety still need further studies to support.
- Nanofat and stromal vascular fraction gel could largely facilitate the application of fat grafting for facial rejuvenation that can be injected intradermally.
- Platelet concentrates, such as platelet-rich plasma and platelet-rich fibrin, have been proposed to combine with facial lipofilling, although the results remain controversial.

INTRODUCTION

Fat grafting has been widely performed for reconstructive or cosmetic purpose around the world, attributed mainly to its rich sources, easy harvesting, and minimal invasiveness as a surgical procedure. It can be arbitrarily divided into 3 categories based on volume needed. The "3 categories" are small-volume fat grafting (<100mL), large-volume fat grafting (100–200 mL) and mega-volume fat grafting (>300 mL). Facial fat grafting is a small-volume procedure (<100 cm^3) and is primarily performed for facial rejuvenation, contouring, or regenerative surgery. The unsatisfying retention rate after fat grafting, however, led to unpredictable outcomes, subsequent multiple procedures, and even complications. A variety of methods have been proposed to enhance the results of facial fat grafting, including several established surgical principles and many possible new techniques. This article primarily summarizes recent scientific studies on standardized techniques for autologous facial fat grafting. In addition, several possible new techniques used in facial fat grafting are reviewed.

SURGICAL PRINCIPLES
Donor Site Selection

There are various donor sites with abundant adipose resources that are easily accessible in the supine position and suitable to harvest for facial lipotransfer, such as abdomen, thigh, flank, abdomen, knee, and buttocks. Until now, there

Disclosure: The authors have nothing to disclose.
[a] Department of Plastic Surgery, Xijing Hospital, Fourth Military Medical University, No. 15 Changle Western Road, Xi'an, Shaanxi, China; [b] Division of Plastic Surgery, University of California Davis Medical Center, 2335 Stockton Boulevard, Suite 6008, Sacramento, CA 95817, USA
* Corresponding authors.
E-mail addresses: yichg@163.com (C.Y.); llpu@ucdavis.edu (L.L.Q.P.)

Clin Plastic Surg 47 (2020) 7–17
https://doi.org/10.1016/j.cps.2019.08.001
0094-1298/20/© 2019 Elsevier Inc. All rights reserved.

has been little evidence of the optimal donor site for fat grafting. But the lower abdomen and inner thigh contain a higher density of adipose-derived stem cells (ADSCs)[1]; in addition, ADSCs isolated from thigh showed more robust adipogenic and angiogenic potential as well as higher expression of peroxisome proliferator-activated receptor $\gamma2$ (PPARγ2) and vascular endothelial growth factor (VEGF) than those from the abdomen.[2] In addition, patients' own characteristics play a critical role on ADSCs concentration, vitality, and functionality; for example, fat grafts harvested from a younger age group in women (<45 years old) show higher viability than older age groups.[3] But considering the release of soluble regenerative-related growth factors, the abdomen may be a slight favorite than the inner thigh because of its higher soluble bio-molecules concentrate. Moreover, the release of growth factors negatively correlated with age whereas the content of stromal vascular fractions (SVFs) and ADSCs showed no statistical significance between abdomen and inner thigh.[4] Therefore, lower abdomen and inner thighs maybe more appropriate to be chosen as better donor sites for facial lipofilling.

Fat Graft Harvesting

The syringe aspiration could be considered a standardized technique of option for facial fat graft harvesting by using back-and-forth movement with a syringe which can mechanically and manually extract adipose tissue. It is especially practicable in facial fat grafting because of the small amount of fat requirement and its relatively less traumatic procedure. Generally, a selected and easy-operating incision could be performed with a no. 11 blade for the infiltration of the aesthetic solution. The tumescent solution is needed and usually infiltrated to the donor site 10 minutes to 15 minutes before adipose extraction for easier and less traumatic fat graft harvesting. It usually contains a low concentration (<0.05%) of epinephrine (for decreasing blood loss and bruising, hematoma, and possibility of fat embolism) and lidocaine (for donor site analgesia or hemostasis) in normal saline or lactated Ringer solution. Then, during fat graft harvesting, a 10-mL or 20-mL Luer Lock syringe is used and connected with a harvesting cannula. Previous research has demonstrated that liposuction by a barbed cannula yields more viable ADSCs than a smooth one without reduction the cell viability of the SVF.[5] In addition, lipoaspiration is better performed within the superficial layer of the subcutaneous tissue because SVF cells are located more in the superficial layer.[6] It should be performed evenly, and uneven changes on the skin surface should be avoided after liposuction. Aspiration should be performed gently with back-and-forth movements of the syringe with a 2-mL space vacuum of negative pressure generated in the syringe. Such lower suction pressure may cause less damage to adipocytes. Lipoaspirates are collected gradually inside the syringe.

Fat Graft Processing

Various approaches have been developed to effectively concentrate aspirated fat before transplantation. Those popular techniques include centrifugation, filtration, washing, and gravity sedimentation. These diverse methods are controversial, however, and respectively focused on the most crucial factors among the regenerative remodeling procedures of fat grafts, such as maximizing the amount of ADSCs, preserving the greatest number of intact adipocytes, and decreasing the chance of contamination.[7] Centrifugation at 1200 g (3000 rpm) for 3 minutes is a commonly used method to process harvested fat grafts, originally proposed by Pu.[8] This process may yield more viable adipocytes with more optimal cellular functions. Further study demonstrated that centrifugation (1200 g, for 3 minutes) increases the density of SVFs proportional to the depth of grafts and more viable adipocytes mainly concentrated on middle and bottom layers. The bottom layer showed a higher tissue retention and a better histologic evaluation than the other 2 layers.[9] Further clinical research has also proved that high-density fat that may yield more satisfying results.[10] Possible mechanisms mainly contribute to its concentrating efficacy of viable cells and decreasing the inflammatory response by removing blood and debris.[11,12]

Harvested fat is transferred into several sterile 10-mL syringes and then carefully placed into a centrifuge symmetrically. After centrifugation in 3000 rpm (approximately 1200 g) for 3 minutes, lipoaspirates within each syringe are divided into 3 layers from top to bottom: top oil layer, middle adipose tissue layer, and bottom fluid portion layer (**Fig. 1**). The top oil layer is decanted from the syringe and the bottom fluid is easily drained. The middle adipose tissue layer also can be divided equally into upper, middle, and lower layers, and the lower layer is primarily chosen and transferred into a 1-mL syringe for a more practicable facial lipotransfer whereas the middle layer of the fat is an alternative choice for further lipofilling (**Fig. 2**). It is better to harvest more adipose tissue that may collect more high-density fat to yield better results for facial lipofilling. Based on the authors'

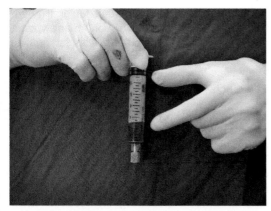

Fig. 1. Harvested fat is centrifuged at 1200 g for 3 minutes and can be divided into 3 layers from top to bottom: oil, pure fat, and fluid. With less trauma during harvesting and centrifugation, less oil component may be expected.

experience, the lower layer is injected for facial volume augmentation whereas the other 2 layers are then prepared as SVF-gel for intradermal injection that may improve the skin quality of the face.

Placement of Fat Grafts

The key to a successful fat graft injection is to achieve an even distribution of fat grafts in the recipient site that may improve the results and reduce the overall complications, such as fat necrosis. Further studies on the mechanisms of fat graft remodeling led to a better understanding of how to place processed fat grafts into the recipient sites, one of the most important techniques in facial lipofilling. The fat grafts should be placed dispersedly, which maximally contact with recipient site to facilitate infiltration of nutrients and

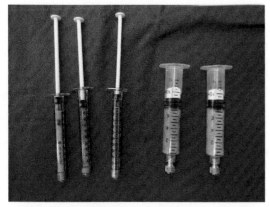

Fig. 2. After centrifugation, pure fat in the midportion of the syringe also can be divided into upper, middle, and lower layers. If possible, only fat from lower layer is selected and used and is transferred to multiple 1-cc syringes for facial fat injection.

neovascularization of fat grafts. A small amount of fat grafts (no more than 0.1 mL) in each pass may improve fat graft survival as well as avoid subsequent complications, such as oil cyst formation, fibrosis, calcification, and even fat embolism.[13] A special device, the microautologous fat transplantation-Gun (MAFT-GUN, Taiwan) has been proposed. It is so delicate that it can inject each parcel volume at 1/60 mL to 1/240 mL.[14] Fat grafts should be injected into multiple bypasses in multiple tissue planes and tunnels. The diameter of injected fat is directly dependent on the diameter of injection cannulas, and the most commonly used cannulas are 5 cm to 9 cm in length with a blunt tip and 1 opening on the side for facial lipofilling. Because the central necrosis of fat grafts may occur by using an injection cannula larger than 14G or injecting more than 0.1 mL in each pass, injecting very tiny volume in each pass and selecting smaller size of cannulas for facial fat grafting should be considred.[15] Recipient site preparation, before facial fat grafting, also may be helpful to enhance the outcomes of lipotransfer. Microneedling has been shown to improve the retention of grafted fat by virtually increasing neovascularization via triggered complex cascade of multiple growth factors.[16] Further studies are necessary to provide more convinced evidences for its clinical application.

Additional Considerations

A recent study proposed that the facial fat compartment plays a crucial role in improving the overall outcomes of facial lipotransfer. Facial fat compartment was first reported by Rohrich and Pessa[17] through an anatomy study and the results found that the subcutaneous fat in the face was partitioned into several independent anatomic facial fat compartments. Those multiple fat compartments are separated by fascial condensations and form an interconnecting framework, which provides a retaining system for the face.[18] Aging-dependent changes are strongly linked to the voluminal changes of facial fat compartments, which a significant volume of deep fat was decreased over time.[19] Knowing these anatomic characteristics would largely help performing a more specifically and more precision preoperative analysis for facial lipotransfer and could subsequently yield more satisfying results for facial rejuvenation.[20,21]

The fat graft site should be immobilized after the first 5 days to 7 days for a better remodeling by taping over the grafted areas. A previous study showed that regional immobilization of the recipient areas may help prevent damage to newly formed vessels and enhance the function of

ADSCs.[22] Therefore, it is also important to inform patients to avoid excessive facial movements during the postoperative recovering period.

POSSIBLE NEW TECHNIQUES FOR FACIAL FAT GRAFTING

With the continuous research on the mechanisms of fat grafting, several novel concepts and techniques have been proposed to enhance the quality and retention after facial fat grafting (**Table 1**). These methods were based primarily on experiments and clinical studies and can be divided into 2 approaches: adding extra components (such as stem cells and platelet concentrates) and fat preparations (such as SVFs, SVF-gel, and nanofat).

The Use of Stem Cells for Facial Fat Grafting

Bone marrow–derived stem cells

Bone marrow–derived stem cells (BMSCs) exhibit self-renewal capacity and multipotency and can be induced to differentiate into multiple cell lineages, such as adipocytes, osteocytes, and chondrocytes.[23] It has been reported that BMSCs participate in the tissue regeneration/remodeling after fat grafting by contributing to form capillary networks and provide new ADSCs.[24] Applying additional fresh BMSCs and expanded BMSCs could improve the outcome of fat grafting, as evidenced by a graft's retention, quality, and neovascularization.[25] It also is indicated that better efficacy has been achieved by using primary compared with expanded BMSCs, possibly because the multiple cell components found in freshly isolated BMSCs but not in homogeneous

expanded BMSCs are important for graft retention. Moreover, cotransfer of bone marrow aspirate/bone marrow concentrate with fat grafting also has been proved a potential preferred choice to enhance the retention of grafted fat in a clinical setting (**Fig. 3**).[26] A further clinical trial has evaluated the applicability of BMSC-assisted fat grafting in patients with Romberg disease and found that it is more effective than conventional facial lipotransfer in terms of fat graft volume retention.[27] This promising method may become the optimal choice for those patients who are thin, with minimal fat available for facial fat grafting. The mechanism of BMSCs enhancing the result of facial lipotransfer is possibly due to their promotion of neovasculogenesis and adipogenesis. The guidelines and standardized procedures for the clinical application of BMSCs, however, specifically those pertaining to their isolation, preparation, and injection and optimal numbers, have not been established, and the long-term safety of BMSCs and the detailed mechanisms remain to be confirmed.

Adipose-derived stem cells

ADSCs were first isolated from human adipose tissue that exhibits characteristics similar to BMSCs, including proliferative self-renewal capacities and multilineage differentiation potential.[28] Considering the abundant stem cell source as well as the simpler and minimally invasive procedures, ADSCs seem more suitable for tissue repair and regeneration than other mesenchymal stem cells. Previous research has proved that adipocytes and ADSCs are categorized into 3 zones (survival, regeneration, and necrosis) after lipotransfer, each

Table 1
Possible new techniques for facial fat grafting

Methods	Mechanism	Clinical Relevance
Stem cells		
ADSCs BMSCs	Directly differentiation ability and paracrine capability	Abundant resources Feasible for slim patients
Fat preparations		
SVFs	Heterogeneous cell population	Clinically feasible
Nanofat	SVF cells without adipocytes	Intradermal injection
SVF-gel	High density of SVF cells and extracellular matrix	Effective for both volumization and rejuvenation
Platelet concentrates		
PRP	Growth factors and plasma	Food and Drug Administration approved
PRF	Growth factors and 3-D fibrin scaffold	Clinically feasible without any exogenous additives
CGF	Growth factors, 3-D fibrin scaffold, and CD34$^+$ cells	The safety and efficacy not yet determined

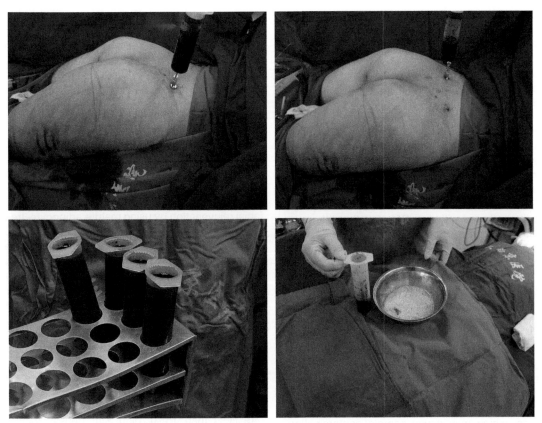

Fig. 3. Processes of BMSCs combined with fat grafting. (*Top left, top right*) Bone marrow is harvested from bilateral iliac bones of each patient; (*bottom left*) bone marrow collection; and (*bottom right*) BMSCs were isolated from bone marrow and fully mixed with prepared autologous fat grafts at a ratio of 1:2 vol/vol.

depending mainly on the distance from the graft surface.[29] Therefore, survived ADSCs may play a key role in stimulating adipogenesis and angiogenesis during regeneration after fat grafting. The efficacy of ex vivo expanded ADSCs has been proved to largely enhance the outcomes of fat grafting in both experimental and clinical contexts, primarily via its directly differentiation (such as adipocytes and endothelial-like cells) and paracrine properties (immunomodulate and inducing angiogenesis).[30–33] In addition, the combination use of ex vivo cultured ADSCs with conventional fat improved the overall clinical results of facial lipofilling in decreasing multiple procedures as well as increasing the satisfaction of patients.[34] Meanwhile, the cultivated ADSCs are time-consuming and may take several weeks. There are several potential problems with using ex vivo ADSCs, such as the increasing risk of contamination and the cost; these issues may limit its clinical applications.[31] Still, further long-term and randomized controlled clinical trials (RCTs) may be necessary to determine the safety and efficacy of ex vivo expanded ADSCs in facial fat grafting. In addition,

the guidelines and standardized procedures for the clinical application of ADSCs, including their indications, have not been established.

The Use of Fat Preparations for Facial Fat Grafting

Cell-assisted lipotransfer and stromal vascular fraction

For more convenient and efficient application of ADSCs, cell-assisted lipotransfer (CAL) has been proposed clinically.[35] Specifically, the lipoaspirate is divided into two parts, one for the preparation of SVF and then SVF was combined with the second part of lipoaspirate (the other part of fat grafts) and transplanted to the recipient site. It is a more time-saving technique by using freshly isolated SVF than ex vivo expanded ADSCs for fat lipofilling. SVF could be directly obtained for the ADSCs supplementation by a collagenase isolation without extra culture. This could largely facilitate the clinical utilization of ADSCs. Until now, several studies have evaluated the effects of CAL in clinical lipotransfer, but the results were not consistent.

Recent systematic reviews have revealed the efficacy (the ability to enhance the retention of grafted fat) and the safety (the incidence of complications and the need for multiple procedures) of CAL used clinically. Eleven articles were involved in facial lipofilling and all of the inclusive studies were evaluated in an objective measurement (computed tomography, magnetic resonance imaging, and 3-dimensional [3-D] measurement). The technique may be suitable for facial lipotransfer because facial CAL may increase the retention rate of fat grafts significantly and avoid the incidences of multiple procedures.[35] Other studies also showed the decreased incidence of the overall complications compared with non-CAL, but the difference was not statistically significant.[36,37] This promising technique seems to be available to overcome the limitations of conventional lipotransfer. Current literature is insufficient, however, to support its routine clinical applications and thus more RCTs with large sample sizes are needed to confirm its efficacy and safety.

Nanofat

Although most of the recent studies have demonstrated the efficacy and the safety of CAL in facial lipotransfer, obtaining SVF still requires extra enzymatic digestions for approximately 40 minutes, which may cause sample contamination and also may raise some ethical concerns. As a consequence, nonenzymatic SVF isolation has been developed to limit collagenase use. In 2013, a novel fat preparation—nanofat—was proposed by Tonnard and colleagues,[38] which not only produces collagenase-free SVF but also makes it possible to inject more superficially with much finer sharp needles. This evolutional technique is actually a type of microfat that does not reach the standard of real nanoscale. It is extracted through a mechanical process that destroys most of the mature adipocytes. In brief, the lipoaspirate is mechanically emulsified and filtered into a liquid suspension (containing SVF and CD34$^+$ cells) that can be injected with finer sharp needles. Its tissue volumization capacity is significantly diminished because of the great reduction of viable adipocytes. It is suitable, however, for tissue revitalization, such as skin rejuvenation, and can be incorporated with conventional lipotransfer for facial rejuvenation.[39,40] Some methods for nanofat improvement have been reported, aiming to enrich the amount and the cytoactive ADSCs via centrifugation of the nanofat.[41,42] Furthermore, a novel device—nanofat needling—has been proposed. It combines microneedling with nanofat injection to facilitate and standardize the delivery of nanofat into the

papillary dermis level.[43] Its clinical applications have shown the improvement of facial rejuvenation by reduction of rhytides and enhancement of skin texture. The mechanisms of this action may mainly contribute to ADSCs that stimulate the production of collagen I proteins and remolded elastic fibers.[43,44]

Stromal vascular fraction gel

ADSCs' density in nanofat is unsatisfactory, however, because of the residual oil component. Furthermore, a previous study has shown that oil drops may cause inflammation during the fat modulation after grafting.[45] Another potential option for facial rejuvenation by using mature adipocyte–free condensed ADSCs product was proposed by Yao and colleagues,[46] known as SVF-gel. But unlike nanofat, SVF-gel eliminates most of the lipid and other undesired components but leaves SVF cells and extracellular matrix behind. The process for preparation is similar to nanofat but a unique flocculation is performed by adding extra 0.5 mL of oil, followed by another centrifugation (2000 g for 3 minutes), and, finally, SVF-gel is extracted from the lower layer (**Fig. 4**). In this way, ADSCs' density could be largely improved and the oil component greatly decreased. This innovative product is defined as follows: low condensing rate (less than 15%), high SVF density (higher than 4.0×10^5 cells/mL), and can be injected through a 27-gauge needle. Preclinical study has demonstrated that grafted SVF-gel modulated fast adipogenesis and angiogenesis as well as rapid infiltration of immune cells at the very early stage of injection, which may contribute to a long-term higher volume retention through a unique regeneration process.[47] Host cell–mediated adipogenesis is observed during the fat remodeling, indicating that adipose tissue also possesses regenerative capabilities not just volumetric filler. A subsequent clinical trial showed better volumization and rejuvenation effects in the SVF-gel group compared with conventional fat grafting with the Coleman technique.[48]

The Use of Platelet Concentrates for Facial Fat Grafting

Rapid neovascularization of fat grafts is another crucial factor to improve the retention and the quality after facial fat grafting. Recently, autologous platelet products have aroused plastic surgeons' interests. Those platelet concentrates (platelet-rich plasma [PRP], platelet-rich fibrin [PRF], and concentrated growth factor [CGF]) have been reported to significantly promote angiogenesis of grafted fat.[49]

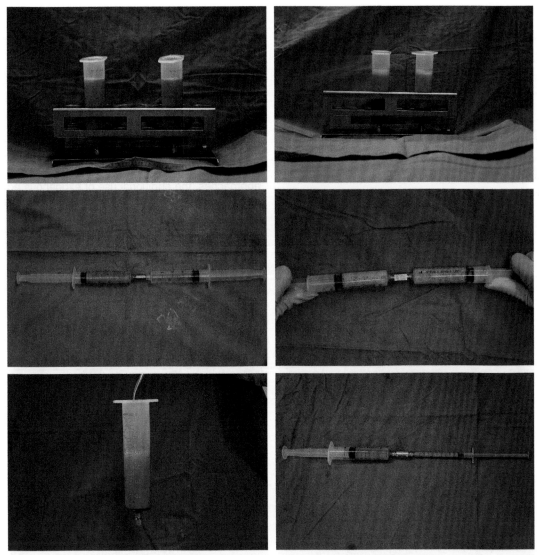

Fig. 4. SVF-gel preparation. (*Top left*) Fat is harvested by Coleman technique; (*top right*) lipoaspirates are then centrifuged at 1200 g for 3 minutes and all of the bottom fluid portion and most of the top oil component are drained out; (*middle left*) isolated fat is then transferred to a sterile 20-mL syringe, which connects with another syringe by a female-to-female Luer lock connector, and mechanically emulsified by shifting these 2 syringes; (*middle right*) the flocculation process is for oil removal; (*bottom left*) mechanically emulsified fat was performed with another centrifugation, at 2000 g for 3 minutes, and SVF-gel is isolated from the middle layer; and (*bottom right*) SVF-gel is transferred to a smaller syringe (1 mL) for further facial injections.

Platelet-rich plasma

PRP contains considerably concentrated platelets, which would release multiple proangiogenic cytokines and growth factors after being activated. Its preparation has not been consistent, but traditionally, it is derived from anticoagulated whole blood through double-spin centrifugation (**Fig. 5**). Many preclinical studies have demonstrated significant improvement of neovascularization after combined PRP with fat grafting, consequently resulting in enhanced tissue retention.[50–52] Possible mechanisms are attributed mainly to its nutrient components, improvements of angiogenesis, and adipogenic differentiation capability to the fat grafts. Most of clinical studies have subsequently indicated the benefits of PRP in improving facial lipofilling by improving fat graft retention and reducing postoperative recovery time.[53,54] Its benefits for volumetric maintenance, however, are still controversial in the current literature. Remarkable differences among studies may are attributed

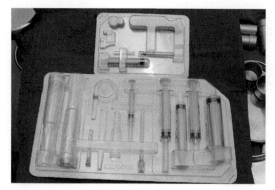

Fig. 5. Device for PRP preparation.

mainly to various methodological factors for evaluation (diverse centrifugation conditions and activation methods) that affect the efficacy of PRP and produce heterogeneous results. Moreover, commercially extraction systems are more likely to be used in clinical settings that makes them even more difficult to evaluate. Nevertheless, several recent RCTs of PRP associated with facial fat grafting have been performed and revealed that PRP did not improve graft retention rates but did accelerate the postoperational recovery.[55,56] In any case, the highly inconsistent methodological approaches, the additional use of exogenous additives, and the releasing speed of growth factors

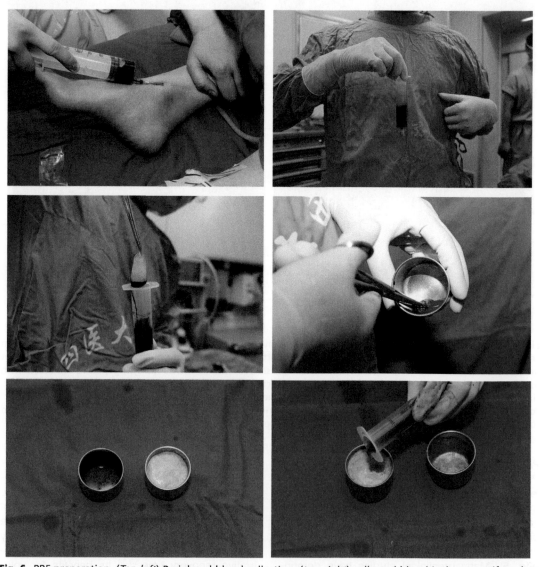

Fig. 6. PRF preparation. (*Top left*) Peripheral blood collection; (*top right*) collected blood is then centrifuged at 2000 rpm for 10 minutes; (*middle left*) PRF is extracted from blood; (*middle right, bottom left*) PRF is cut into approximately 1 mm³ pieces; and (*bottom right*) PRF granules are mixed with prepared fat at a ratio of 1:2 vol/vol.

along with the optimal ratio of PRP to fat grafts must be determined by further studies.

Platelet-rich fibrin and concentrated growth factor

PRF is considered a new generation of platelet concentrates, which are less expensive, easier to operate, and more convenient than PRP and can be directly obtained in a single centrifugation step (3000 rpm for 10 minutes) without adding any anticoagulants or activators. It is feasible for plastic surgeons to perform it in a clinical setting (**Fig. 6**). This transient anticoagulant-free extraction forms a special 3-D fibrin structure, which could subsequently capture concentrated platelets and growth factors and contribute to a gradual and long-term release of angiogenic growth factors and cytokines. Also, the compact fibrin scaffold provides a suitable microenvironment for the adipogenic and angiogenic activity of postgrafting remodeling. Theoretically, PRF would be superior to PRP for facial fat grafting in a clinical setting.[57,58] A recent animal study compared the efficacy between PRP and PRF in fat grafting and found that PRF combined with lipoinjection improved tissue retention and quality of the grafted fat compared with control group. Further histologic evaluations showed a higher vessel density compared with the PRP-treated and control groups.[59] Keyhan and colleagues[60] reported a self-controlled clinical trial of cotransplanting PRF or PRP with autologous fat grafts for facial lipofilling. One year later, the results indicated that PRF may be more effective than PRP in facial lipotransfer and that the absorption rate was lower in fat + PRF side by comparing presurgical and postsurgical photographic views.[61] CGF is another type of platelet concentrate that is obtained from a special commercial centrifugal device via a series of centrifugation without adding any exogenous additives, containing CD34+ cells and a thick fibrin matrix.[62] It also may improve the results of fat grafting.[63] More well-designed randomized clinical trials are needed to prove its efficacy in facial fat grafting.

SUMMARY

Facial fat grafting can be performed with a more standardized technique based on many valid scientific studies with good and consistent results by many experienced surgeons for facial rejuvenation, contouring, and regenerative surgery. Nanofat grafting has recently been reported in the literature and can be performed in patients for additional benefits, such as enhanced skin rejuvenation, in addition to the more established and standardized technique. Additives, such as stem cells (BMSCs and ADSCs), fat preparations (SVF, nanofat, and SVF-gel), and platelet concentrates (PRP, PRF, and CGF), may improve the survival after fat grafting but RCTs are needed to determine their safety and efficacy as well as clinical indications for each technique.

REFERENCES

1. Padoin AV, Braga-Silva J, Martins P, et al. Sources of processed lipoaspirate cells: influence of donor site on cell concentration. Plast Reconstr Surg 2008;122: 614–8.
2. Li W, Zhang Y, Chen C, et al. Increased angiogenic and adipogenic differentiation potentials in adipose-derived stromal cells from thigh subcutaneous adipose depots compared with cells from the abdomen. Aesthet Surg J 2019;39:P140–9.
3. Geissler PJ, Davis K, Roostaeian J, et al. Improving fat transfer viability: the role of aging, body mass index, and harvest site. Plast Reconstr Surg 2014;134: 227–32.
4. Grasys J, Kim BS, Pallua N. Content of soluble factors and characteristics of stromal vascular fraction cells in lipoaspirates from different subcutaneous adipose tissue depots. Aesthet Surg J 2016;36: 831–41.
5. Caggiati A, Germani A, Di Carlo A, et al. Naturally adipose stromal cell-enriched fat graft: comparative polychromatic flow cytometry study of fat harvested by barbed or blunt multihole cannula. Aesthet Surg J 2017;37:591–602.
6. Di Taranto G, Cicione C, Visconti G, et al. Qualitative and quantitative differences of adipose-derived stromal cells from superficial and deep subcutaneous lipoaspirates: a matter of fat. Cytotherapy 2015;17: 1076–89.
7. Cleveland EC, Albano NJ, Hazen A. Roll, spin, wash, or filter? Processing of lipoaspirate for autologous fat grafting: an updated, evidence-based review of the literature. Plast Reconstr Surg 2015;136:706–13.
8. Pu LLQ, Coleman SR, Cui X, et al. Autologous fat grafts harvested and refined by the coleman technique: a comparative study. Plast Reconstr Surg 2008;122:932–7.
9. Qiu L, Su Y, Zhang D, et al. Identification of the centrifuged lipoaspirate fractions suitable for postgrafting survival. Plast Reconstr Surg 2016;137: 67e–76e.
10. De Francesco F, Guastafierro A, Nicoletti G, et al. The selective centrifugation ensures a better in vitro isolation of ASCs and restores a soft tissue regeneration in vivo. Int J Mol Sci 2017;18:1038.
11. Salinas HM, Broelsch GF, Fernandes JR, et al. Comparative analysis of processing methods in fat grafting. Plast Reconstr Surg 2014;134:675–83.

12. Streit L, Jaros J, Sedlakova V, et al. A comprehensive in vitro comparison of preparation techniques for fat grafting. Plast Reconstr Surg 2017;139:670e–82e.

13. Liu S, Chen X, Su Y, et al. Association of autologous fat injection in facial artery with ophthalmological complications: an experimental animal study. JAMA Facial Plast Surg 2018;20:445.

14. Chou CK, Lee SS, Lin TY, et al. Micro-autologous fat transplantation (MAFT) for forehead volumizing and contouring. Aesthetic Plast Surg 2017;41:845–55.

15. James IB, Bourne DA, DiBernardo G, et al. The architecture of fat grafting II. Plast Reconstr Surg 2018;142:1219–25.

16. Sezgin B, Ozmen S, Bulam H, et al. Improving fat graft survival through preconditioning of the recipient site with microneedling. J Plast Reconstr Aesthet Surg 2014;67:712–20.

17. Rohrich RJ, Pessa JE. The fat compartments of the face: anatomy and clinical implications for cosmetic surgery. Plast Reconstr Surg 2007;119:2219–27, 2228-2231.

18. Rohrich RJ, Pessa JE. The retaining system of the face: histologic evaluation of the septal boundaries of the subcutaneous fat compartments. Plast Reconstr Surg 2008;121:1804–9.

19. Gierloff M, Stohring C, Buder T, et al. Aging changes of the midfacial fat compartments: a computed tomographic study. Plast Reconstr Surg 2012;129:263–73.

20. Denadai R, Buzzo CL, Raposo-Amaral CA, et al. Facial contour symmetry outcomes after site-specific facial fat compartment augmentation with fat grafting in facial deformities. Plast Reconstr Surg 2019;143:544–56.

21. Wang W, Xie Y, Huang RL, et al. Facial contouring by targeted restoration of facial fat compartment volume: the midface. Plast Reconstr Surg 2017;139:563–72.

22. Shi N, Guo S, Su Y, et al. Improvement in the retention rate of transplanted fat in muscle by denervation. Aesthet Surg J 2018;38:1026–34.

23. Wang Y, Chen X, Cao W, et al. Plasticity of mesenchymal stem cells in immunomodulation: pathological and therapeutic implications. Nat Immunol 2014;15:1009–16.

24. Doi K, Ogata F, Eto H, et al. Differential contributions of graft-derived and host-derived cells in tissue regeneration/remodeling after fat grafting. Plast Reconstr Surg 2015;135:1607–17.

25. Zhao J, Yi C, Zheng Y, et al. Enhancement of fat graft survival by bone marrow-derived mesenchymal stem cell therapy. Plast Reconstr Surg 2013;132:1149–57.

26. Xing W, Mu D, Wang Q, et al. Improvement of fat graft survival with autologous bone marrow aspirate and bone marrow concentrate: a one-step method. Plast Reconstr Surg 2016;137:676e–86e.

27. Jianhui Z, Chenggang Y, Binglun L, et al. Autologous fat graft and bone marrow–derived mesenchymal stem cells assisted fat graft for treatment of parry-romberg syndrome. Ann Plast Surg 2014;73: S99–103.

28. Bacakova L, Zarubova J, Travnickova M, et al. Stem cells: their source, potency and use in regenerative therapies with focus on adipose-derived stem cells - a review. Biotechnol Adv 2018;36:1111–26.

29. Mashiko T, Yoshimura K. How does fat survive and remodel after grafting? Clin Plast Surg 2015;42: 181–90.

30. Philips BJ, Grahovac TL, Valentin JE, et al. Prevalence of endogenous CD34+ adipose stem cells predicts human fat graft retention in a xenograft model. Plast Reconstr Surg 2013;132:845–58.

31. Kolle SF, Fischer-Nielsen A, Mathiasen AB, et al. Enrichment of autologous fat grafts with ex-vivo expanded adipose tissue-derived stem cells for graft survival: a randomised placebo-controlled trial. Lancet 2013;382:1113–20.

32. Chen X, Yan L, Guo Z, et al. Adipose-derived mesenchymal stem cells promote the survival of fat grafts via crosstalk between the Nrf2 and TLR4 pathways. Cell Death Dis 2016;7:e2369.

33. Hong KY, Yim S, Kim HJ, et al. The fate of the adipose-derived stromal cells during angiogenesis and adipogenesis after cell-assisted lipotransfer. Plast Reconstr Surg 2018;141:365–75.

34. Bashir MM, Sohail M, Bashir A, et al. Outcome of conventional adipose tissue grafting for contour deformities of face and role of ex vivo expanded adipose tissue-derived stem cells in treatment of such deformities. J Craniofac Surg 2018;29: 1143–7.

35. Matsumoto D, Sato K, Gonda K, et al. Cell-assisted lipotransfer: supportive use of human adipose-derived cells for soft tissue augmentation with lipoinjection. Tissue Eng 2006;12:3375–82.

36. Zhou Y, Wang J, Li H, et al. Efficacy and safety of cell-assisted lipotransfer: a systematic review and meta-analysis. Plast Reconstr Surg 2016;137: 44e–57e.

37. Laloze J, Varin A, Gilhodes J, et al. Cell-assisted lipotransfer: friend or foe in fat grafting? Systematic review and meta-analysis. J Tissue Eng Regen Med 2018;12:e1237–50.

38. Tonnard P, Verpaele A, Peeters G, et al. Nanofat grafting: basic research and clinical applications. Plast Reconstr Surg 2013;132:1017–26.

39. Mashiko T, Wu SH, Feng J, et al. Mechanical micronization of lipoaspirates: squeeze and emulsification techniques. Plast Reconstr Surg 2017;139:79–90.

40. Yu Q, Cai Y, Huang H, et al. Co-transplantation of nanofat enhances neovascularization and fat graft survival in nude mice. Aesthet Surg J 2018;38: 667–75.

41. Zheng H, Qiu L, Su Y, et al. Conventional nanofat and SVF/ADSC-Concentrated nanofat: a comparative study on improving photoaging of nude mice skin. Aesthet Surg J 2019. [Epub ahead of print].

42. Pallua N, Grasys J, Kim BS. Enhancement of progenitor cells by two-step centrifugation of emulsified lipoaspirates. Plast Reconstr Surg 2018;142:99–109.

43. Verpaele A, Tonnard P, Jeganathan C, et al. Nanofat needling: a novel method for uniform delivery of adipose-derived stromal vascular fraction into the skin. Plast Reconstr Surg 2019;143:1062–5.

44. Uyulmaz S, Sanchez MN, Rezaeian F, et al. Nanofat grafting for scar treatment and skin quality improvement. Aesthet Surg J 2018;38:421–8.

45. Kato H, Mineda K, Eto H, et al. Degeneration, regeneration, and cicatrization after fat grafting: dynamic total tissue remodeling during the first 3 months. Plast Reconstr Surg 2014;133:303e–13e.

46. Yao Y, Dong Z, Liao Y, et al. Adipose extracellular matrix/stromal vascular fraction gel: a novel adipose tissue-derived injectable for stem cell therapy. Plast Reconstr Surg 2017;139:867–79.

47. Zhang Y, Cai J, Zhou T, et al. Improved long-term volume retention of stromal vascular fraction gel grafting with enhanced angiogenesis and adipogenesis. Plast Reconstr Surg 2018;141:676e–86e.

48. Yao Y, Cai J, Zhang P, et al. Adipose stromal vascular fraction gel grafting: a new method for tissue volumization and rejuvenation. Dermatol Surg 2018;44:1278–86.

49. Xiong S, Qiu L, Zhao J, et al. The role of platelet concentrates in facial fat grafting. Ann Plast Surg 2018; 81:S117–23.

50. Seyhan N, Alhan D, Ural AU, et al. The effect of combined use of platelet-rich plasma and adipose-derived stem cells on fat graft survival. Ann Plast Surg 2015;74:615–20.

51. Li F, Guo W, Li K, et al. Improved fat graft survival by different volume fractions of platelet-rich plasma and adipose-derived stem cells. Aesthet Surg J 2015;35: 319–33.

52. Zhou S, Chang Q, Lu F, et al. Injectable mussel-inspired immobilization of platelet-rich plasma on microspheres bridging adipose micro-tissues to improve autologous fat transplantation by controlling release of PDGF and VEGF, angiogenesis, stem cell migration. Adv Healthc Mater 2017;6. https://doi.org/10.1002/adhm.201700131.

53. Willemsen JCN, van der Lei B, Vermeulen KM, et al. The effects of platelet-rich plasma on recovery time and aesthetic outcome in facial rejuvenation: preliminary retrospective observations. Aesthet Plast Surg 2014;38:1057–63.

54. Sasaki GH. A Preliminary clinical trial comparing split treatments to the face and hand with autologous fat grafting and platelet-rich plasma (PRP): a 3D, IRB-approved study. Aesthet Surg J 2019;39: 675–86.

55. Fontdevila J, Guisantes E, Martínez E, et al. Double-blind clinical trial to compare autologous fat grafts versus autologous fat grafts with PDGF. Plast Reconstr Surg 2014;134:219e–30e.

56. Willemsen J, Van Dongen J, Spiekman M, et al. The addition of platelet-rich plasma to facial lipofilling: a double-blind, placebo-controlled, randomized trial. Plast Reconstr Surg 2018;141:331–43.

57. Al-Chalabi N, Al-Quisi AF, Abdul LT. Single session facial lipostructure by using autologous fat mixed with platelet-rich fibrin injected by using facial autologous muscular injection technique. J Craniofac Surg 2018;29:e267–71.

58. Yu P, Zhai Z, Jin X, et al. Clinical application of platelet-rich fibrin in plastic and reconstructive surgery: a systematic review. Aesthet Plast Surg 2018;42:511–9.

59. Xiong S, Qiu L, Su Y, et al. Platelet-rich plasma and platelet-rich fibrin enhance the outcomes of fat grafting: a comparative study. Plast Reconstr Surg 2019; 143:1201e–12e.

60. Keyhan S, Hemmat S, Badri A, et al. Use of platelet-rich fibrin and platelet-rich plasma in combination with fat graft: which is more effective during facial lipostructure? J Oral Maxillofac Surg 2013;71: 610–21.

61. Liao HT, Marra KG, Rubin JP. Application of platelet-rich plasma and platelet-rich fibrin in fat grafting: basic science and literature review. Tissue Eng Part B Rev 2014;20:267–76.

62. Rodella LF, Favero G, Boninsegna R, et al. Growth factors, CD34 positive cells, and fibrin network analysis in concentrated growth factors fraction. Microsc Res Tech 2011;74:772–7.

63. Hu Y, Jiang Y, Wang M, et al. Concentrated growth factor enhanced fat graft survival: a comparative study. Dermatol Surg 2018;44:976–84.

Fat Grafting for Facial Rejuvenation
My Preferred Approach

Lee L.Q. Pu, MD, PhD

KEYWORDS

- Fat transplantation • Fat grafting • Lipotransfer • Coleman technique • Facial rejuvenation

KEY POINTS

- The preferred donor sites for fat grafting should be the lower abdomen or inner thigh.
- Fat grafts should be harvested with low negative pressure to ensure the integrity and viability of adipocytes.
- Fat grafts can be processed with proper centrifugation that can reliably produce purified fat and concentrated growth factors and adipose-derived stem cells.
- Preinjection of local anesthetic with epinephrine to planned fat grafting sites prevents intravascular injections and possible fat embolism.
- Fat grafts should be injected with gentle injection of a tiny amount per pass in multiple tissue planes and levels and with multiple passes to ensure maximal contact of the graft with vascularized tissue in the recipient site.

INTRODUCTION

Fat grafting is considered an excellent option for facial rejuvenation because fat is abundant, readily available, inexpensive, host compatible, and can be harvested easily and repeatedly.[1] Compared with any available synthetic filler, fat can be an ideal filler for facial rejuvenation because the clinical result after fat grafting can be permanent without any concerns or complications related to fillers.[2] However, the overall survival rate after fat grafting may still be less optimal. To improve fat graft survival has therefore been constantly the driving force for clinicians to search for better techniques of fat grafting.

Since mid-1990s, Dr Sydney R. Coleman from New York City has championed and popularized the technique primarily for facial fat grafting. His technique, also referred to as the Coleman technique, emphasizes proper harvest, process, and placement of fat grafts.[3–5]

For the last 10 years, fat grafting has become a popular procedure in plastic surgery, especially for facial rejuvenation either with or without other surgical procedures. In this article, the author introduces his preferred and more scientifically sound technique for fat grafting to the face. He also describes why each step should be performed based on most recent scientific studies by many investigators. Several case examples are presented to highlight those important principles in facial fat grafting.

PREOPERATIVE EVALUATION AND SPECIAL CONSIDERATIONS

Each patient's general health and past medical or surgical history should be reviewed first.

Disclosure: The author has nothing to disclose.
Division of Plastic Surgery, University of California Davis, 2335 Stockton Boulevard, Suite 6008, Sacramento, CA 95817, USA
E-mail address: llpu@ucdavis.edu

Clin Plastic Surg 47 (2020) 19–29
https://doi.org/10.1016/j.cps.2019.08.002

Concerns about his or her facial aging from each patient should carefully be evaluated. The quality of facial skin and the anatomy of the face, including symmetry, signs of facial aging such as excess skin, ptosis of structures, prominent lines, and soft tissue atrophy in certain anatomic areas, are analyzed and documented. The potential donor sites for fat graft harvest are also examined. The detailed plan for facial fat grafting can be formulated and communicated with the patient.

Anesthesia for harvest of fat grafts can be performed under general anesthesia or local anesthesia with intravenous sedation. The tumescent solution used for donor site analgesia or hemostasis should contain the lowest concentration of lidocaine possible because its high concentration may have detrimental effect on the adipocyte function and viability.[6] In general, the author uses 0.03% of lidocaine in 1 L of Ringer lactate solution. The tumescent solution also contains epinephrine with a concentration of 1:200,000. Epinephrine can precipitate vasoconstriction in the donor sites as well as the recipient sites, which may decrease blood loss, bruising, hematoma, and the possibility of intraarterial injection of the transplanted fat especially when injecting around periorbital or temporal area.

Whether overcorrection is necessary or not for fat grafting remains unclear. Because the viable fat grafts are only observed in the peripheral zone approximately 1.5 mm from the edge of the grafts and the percentage of graft viability depends on its thickness and geometric shape,[7] overcorrection for "better" graft survival in the recipient site seems to be lack of scientific support. In addition, significant overcorrection may increase the incidence of fat necrosis and subsequent calcification or even severe infection.[8] Therefore, "significant" overcorrection should be avoided until its necessity and safety can be confirmed by future studies.

Because overall take rate of fat grafting by even experienced surgeons ranges from 50% to 80%,[1,9,10] additional procedures are always necessary to achieve an optimal outcome. However, there is no scientific study that has addressed the timing of subsequent fat grafting. So far, only one "expert" opinion has been mentioned in the literature regarding this specific issue[11]: "the timing of additional fat grafting sessions should be deferred until 6 months postoperatively to diminish the "inflammatory response" in the grafted area."

It is often difficult to assess the surgical outcome during the first few weeks after fat grafting. In general, the extent of swelling and the waiting period that it needs to resolve is also volume dependent. It has been observed that the transplanted fat gradually loses its volume with time and usually becomes stabilized at 3 months postoperatively if surgical recovery is uneventful. Therefore, the timing of a subsequent fat grafting procedure should be deferred to at least 3 months after previous transplantation.

SURGICAL PROCEDURES
Donor Site Selection

As a rule, donor sites are selected that enhance body contour and are easily accessible in the supine position, which is the position that is used for almost all facial fat grafting procedures. Although there is no evidence of a favorable donor site for harvest of fat grafts because the viability of adipocytes within the fat grafts from different donor sites may be considered equal, higher concentration of adipose-derived stem cells (ADSCs) is found in the lower abdomen and inner thigh in one study.[12] In addition, in younger age group (<45 years old), fat grafts harvested from both lower abdomen and inner thigh have higher viability based on a single assay test.[13] With what is known about the potential role of ADSCs in fat grafting,[14] the lower abdomen and inner thighs should, therefore, be chosen as the "better" donor sites for fat grafting to the face[12,13](**Fig. 1**). These donor sites are not only easily accessible by the surgeons with a patient in the supine position but also scientifically sound as long as patients have adequate amount of adipose tissue in those areas. In the author's practice, a total of 30 cc is usually needed for most facial rejuvenation cases.

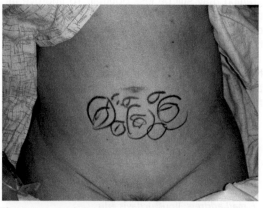

Fig. 1. Lower abdomen is a commonly selected donor site for facial fat grafting.

Fat Grafting Harvesting

The syringe aspiration, as a relatively less traumatic method for harvest of fat grafts, is supported by the more recent studies and should be considered as a standardized technique of choice for harvest of fat grafts.[15] However, this technique can be time consuming even for experienced surgeons and the large quantity of fat grafts may not easily be obtained with this technique.

Placement of incisions can be done with a No. 11 blade in the locations where the future scar can easily be concealed. The size of incision is about 2 to 3 mm. A small clamp is used to dilate the underlying subcutaneous tissue through the incision to allow insertion of the harvesting cannula with ease. The aesthetic solution is then infiltrated to the donor site 10 to 15 minutes before fat extraction, which makes harvesting of fat graft easier and less traumatic. The tip of the infiltration cannula is usually blunt and has one opening on the side. The ratio of aspirated fat to tumescent solution should be about 1:1 so that each pass of fat extraction can be more efficient.

A 10 cc Luer lock syringe is used and connected with a harvesting cannula. For harvesting fat grafts from the lower abdomen or inner thigh, a newly designed harvesting cannula with multiple side holes is used (**Fig. 2**). This kind of cannula can be more efficient for fat extraction. A gentle pull back on the plunger creates a 2 cc space vacuum negative pressure in the syringe. With gentle back and forth movement of the syringe, the fat is gradually collected inside the syringe (**Fig. 3**). After harvest, all incision sites are closed with interrupted sutures once excess tumescent fluid or blood is milked out.

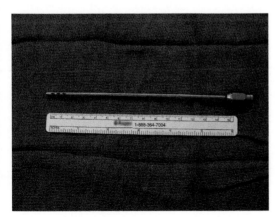

Fig. 2. A newly designed cannula with multiple side holes for fat graft harvest. The cannula has a total of 6 side holes and is quite speedy for fat harvest.

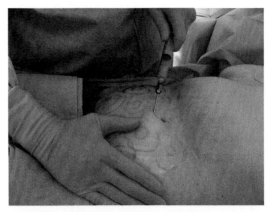

Fig. 3. Fat grafts are aspirated with back and forth movement with a 10 cc syringe and a 2 cm space vacuum negative pressure.

Fat Graft Processing

Several methods have been proposed to effectively remove the infiltrated solution and cell debris within the lipoaspirates and to obtain more concentrated fat grafts. However, it is the most controversial and disagreeable issue in fat grafting even among many experts in the field. Common methods for processing fat grafts include centrifugation, filtration, or gravity sedimentation.

Centrifugation, as proposed by Coleman, is the author's preferred method to process fat grafts. There are several advantages of centrifugation of fat grafts. More viable adipocytes are found at the bottom of middle layer after centrifugation even with a force of 50 g for 2 minutes base on viable cell counts, and this makes manipulation of fat graft for use easier but with better viability.[16,17] Recent studies have shown that proper centrifugation can concentrate not only on adipocytes and ADSCs but also on several angiogenic growth factors within the processed fat grafts.[18,19] Because higher content of stem cell or angiogenic growth factor positively correlated with fat graft survival both in experimental and clinical studies,[20] centrifugation at 3000 rpm (about 1200 g) for 3 minutes seems to offer more benefits for this effectively concentrating adipocytes and ADSCs and should be a valid method of choice for processing fat grafts, especially for small volume fat grafting.[15]

The Luer lock aperture of the 10 cc syringe locked with a plug at completion of harvest is ready for centrifugation (**Fig. 4**). After careful removal of the plunger, all lipoaspirate-filled 10 cc syringes are placed into a centrifuge and are then centrifuged with 3000 rpm (about 1200 g) for 3 minutes. Greater g-force or longer

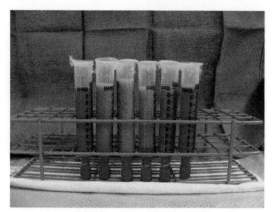

Fig. 4. At completion of fat harvest, each syringe is locked with a plug and covered with a transparent film dressing to prevent prolonged exposure to air and possible contamination. It is ready for centrifugation.

duration of centrifugation may be harmful to adipocytes and is therefore not recommended.[21]

Attention should be made to avoid prolonged exposure of fat grafts to air and to avoid bacterial contamination. After being centrifuged, lipoaspirates with the syringe are divided into 3 layers: the oil content in the upper layer, fatty tissue in the middle layer, and the fluid portion at the bottom (**Fig. 5**). The oil can be decanted from the Luer lock syringe. The residual oil is wicked with a cotton strip or swab. The fluid at the bottom can be easily drained out once the plug at the Luer lock aperture is removed.

The concentrated fat in the syringe can then be transferred to a 1 cc syringe (preferred size of syringe for fat injection to the face) via an adaptor. A 1 cc syringe is made of acrylic material and

has little resistance while fat grafts are injected. In addition, the injected volume can easily be controlled by the surgeon with such a syringe (**Fig. 6**).

Preparation of Recipient Site

Unlike other parts of the body such as breast, pre-expansion to the face for facial rejuvenation is usually not required. Because of rich blood supply in the face, the possibility of intravascular injections causing fat embolism to the brain or eye can be real and may be avoided by preinjection of 1% lidocaine with 1:200,000 epinephrine to planned fat grafting sites for possible vasoconstriction especially in the temporal and periorbital areas. Adequate compression to those areas after injection of abovementioned anesthetic solution is needed in order to minimize swelling in the area so that precise placement of fat grafts can still be made by the surgeon according to the volume requirement of fat grafts in each area. In addition, release firm attachment of the skin over the proposed injected areas such as in the nasolabial fold with a sharp cannula can also be performed so that the space is created between the skin and underlining tissue for placement of fat grafts (**Fig. 7**).

Injection of Fat Grafts

One of the most important techniques of fat grating may be how to inject fat grafts. The key to a successful fat graft injection is to achieve an even distribution of fat grafts in the recipient site. By doing so, the injected fat grafts may have a maximal amount of contact with the tissue in the recipient site for better fat graft survival through plasmatic imbibition and neovascularization

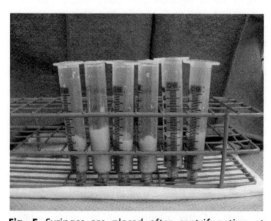

Fig. 5. Syringes are placed after centrifugation at 3000 rpm for 3 minutes. Oil in the upper layer and liquid in the lower layer are discarded. Only the fat grafts in the middle layer are collected.

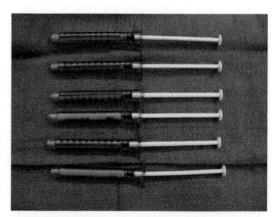

Fig. 6. Fat grafts are transferred to multiple 1 cc syringes for injection. A 1 cc acrylic syringe is preferred for facial fat grafting.

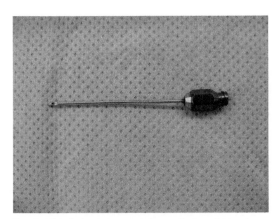

Fig. 7. The forked-tip cannula can be used to release fibrotic tissue, scar, or adhesion.

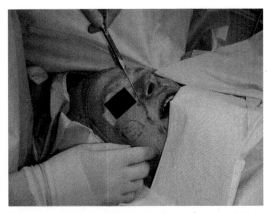

Fig. 9. An intraoperative view shows fat injection to the face. The injection should be meticulously performed based on the techniques described in the article.

(**Fig. 8**). Not only grafting with small volume in each pass can get better surgical outcomes but also complications such as fibrosis, oil cyst formation, calcification, or even infection with large bolus grafting can be avoided. To achieve this goal, small volume (no more than 0.1 cc) of fat grafts should be injected in each pass. Slow injection of 0.5 to -1 cc per second during the withdrawal phase in each pass minimizes trauma to the fat graft.[9,22] Fat grafts should be placed via multiple passes within multiple tissue planes and tunnels in multiple directions[1,9] (**Fig. 9**). The volume requirement for each area of the face in the author's practice is summarized in **Box 1**.

Injection should be as gentle as possible to avoid a possible injury to vessel or nerve. Injection with resistance would compromise the result and increase the chance of associated complications (**Fig. 10**). Only a dull tip injection cannula is selected to avoid accidental intravascular injection (**Fig. 11**). The most commonly used cannulas are 5

Box 1
Volume requirement of fat grafting for each area of the face

Forehead	10–15 cc
Temporal fossa	4–6 cc
Upper eyelid	1 cc
Lower eyelid/cheek junction	1–2 cc
Cheek	4–10 cc
Nasal dorsum	2–4 cc
Nasolabial fold	1–2 cc
Upper/lower lip	1–2 cc
Marionette line	1–2 cc
Chin	4–6 cc

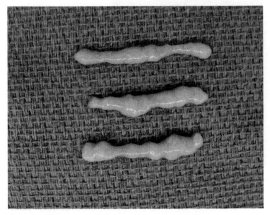

Fig. 8. An example of well-processed and concentrated fat grafts without oils and red blood cells.

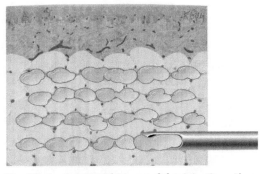

Fig. 10. A proper technique of fat injection. Placement of minuscule amounts of fat grafts with each pass as the cannula is withdrawn. Fat grafts should be placed with multiple bypasses but in multiple tissue planes and tunnels. (*From* Coleman S., et al. Fat Injection from Filling to Regeneration. Thieme New York 2018; with permission.)

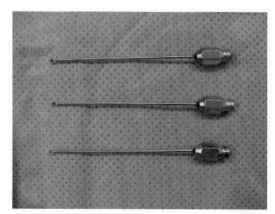

Fig. 11. Several dull tip injection cannulas are used for facial fat grafting.

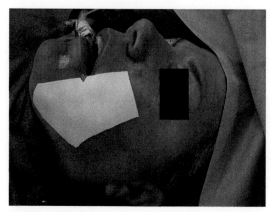

Fig. 12. Taping the injected area for immediate postoperative care after facial fat grafting.

to 9 cm in length and 1 mm in diameter for facial procedure. In general, a smaller cannula should be used for fat grafting to the area such as the periorbital region where only a smaller volume of fat

grafts is injected in each pass. Smaller cannulas may also allow the surgeon to have more precise control over the volume when extremely tiny amount of fat grafts is injected. The cannula

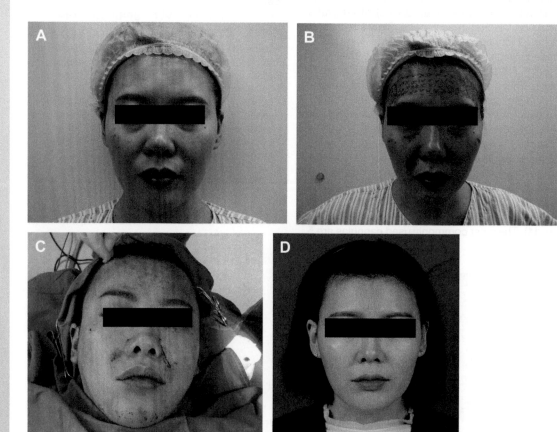

Fig. 13. (*A*) A 29-year-old Asian woman desired facial rejuvenation and contouring. (*B*) The preoperative design and plan for her facial rejuvenation and contouring. (*C*) An immediate intraoperative appearance after her facial fat grafting. She had a total of 37 cc fat grafting to her face (forehead: 15 cc; temporal fossa: 5 cc for each side; medial lid/cheek junction: 1.5 cc for each side; nasolabial fold: 2 cc for each side; and chin: 5 cc). (*D*) The results at 5-month follow-up.

includes straight or curved one and blunt or forked tip in order to meet different needs. The cannula with forked tip can cut through tissues and can be used to release fibrotic tissue or scar, adhesion, or ligament attachments.

Preoperative photograph with a detail planning marked on the patient is important for intraoperative comparison, because the changes need to be made with fat grafting in the operating room usually are very subtle. The surgeon should

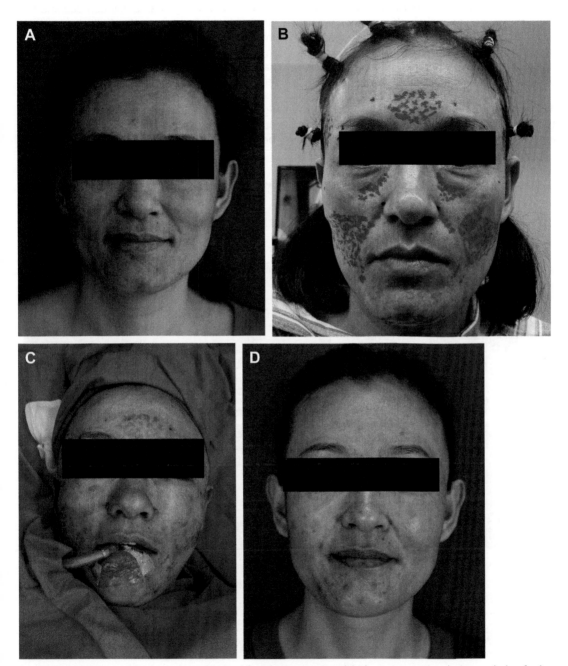

Fig. 14. (*A*) A 42-year-old Asian woman desired facial rejuvenation. (*B*) The preoperative design and plan for her facial rejuvenation. (*C*) An immediate intraoperative appearance after her facial fat grafting. She had a total of 36.8 cc fat grafting to her face (glabella: 2 cc; temporal fossa: 4 cc for right side and 3 cc to left side; upper eyelid: 0.5 cc for each side; medial lower eyelid/cheek junction: 1 cc for each side; nasolabial fold: 1 cc for each side; cheek: 9 cc for right side and 6 cc for left side; perioral: 1 cc for right side and 0.8 cc for left side; and chin: 6 cc). (*D*) The results at 12-month follow-up.

make sure where the cannula tip is during the entire injection process. If there is any doubt about the tip location, tent the cannula tip toward the skin and then see blanching of the skin overlying the advanced cannula to reveal its exact location. If fat grafts are placed in a correct location, the "augmented" effect in the grafted area can easily be identified. If volume is not increased even though grafting is in the right place, other factors that may restrict volume enlargement should be taken into consideration such as fibrotic adhesion or tight skin envelope. Fibrosis or adhesion can be dissected with an 18 gauge needle or a forked tip cannula. Attention should be made to avoid a "bolus" injection, and the basic principles for fat injection should be followed to ensure the better outcome and avoid fat necrosis.

POSTOPERATIVE CARE

Swelling in the recipient site is expected for 1 or 2 weeks and the grafted areas can become firm or hard in the first few weeks. Patients should be informed about this normal process after fat grafting and some reassurance to them may be necessary. However, when fat grafting is done to the face, prolonged swelling (up to 6 weeks) may be expected. During the recovery time, ice packing, tight compression with elastic bandage, or massage in the grafted area should be avoided because all the above may compromise fat graft

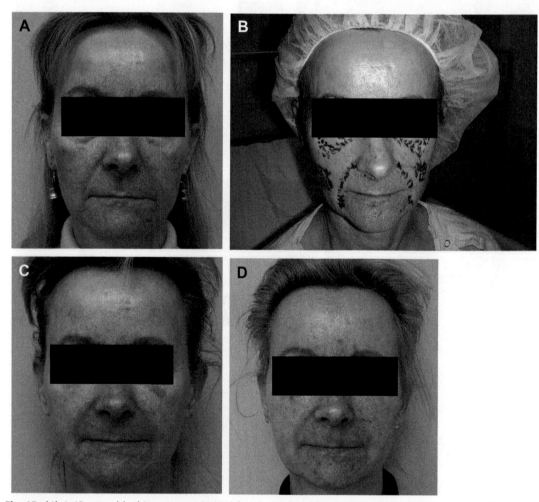

Fig. 15. (*A*) A 42-year-old white woman desired facial and periorbital rejuvenation. (*B*) The preoperative design and plan for her facial and periorbital rejuvenation with fat grafting. She had a total of 15 cc fat grafts to her periorbital area and face (lower eyelid/cheek junction: 1.5 cc for each side; cheek: 3 cc for each side; nasolabial fold: 2 cc for each side; and perioral: 1 cc for each side). She also had bilateral upper and lower blepharoplasty and lateral canthopexy. (*C*) The results at 5 weeks after her facial fat grafting and periorbital procedures. (*D*) The results at 13-month follow-up.

survival and final outcome. However, taping over the grafted areas may relieve some discomfort from swelling and prevent the patient from pressing or touching the areas (**Fig. 12**). Any direct trauma or shear force over the grafted areas may jeopardize fat graft survival and should be avoided.

EXPECTED OUTCOME AND MANAGEMENT OF COMPLICATIONS

Complications of fat grafting to the face are not common and can usually be avoided with meticulous surgery.[3,4] Complications from the donor site are the same as those expected from liposuction, which include depression and uneven body surface. Liposuction for graft harvest should aim to enhance lower abdominal or inner thigh contour by careful assessment for the location of the excess fat. The recipient site may develop

hematoma, infection, nerve injury, or rarely, vessel thrombosis as the acute complications or small fat necrosis as the late complications. Fortunately, acute complications are rare and usually do not develop if the procedure is performed by experienced surgeons. Fat necrosis may develop continued fibrosis from the macrophages trying to phagocytose the nonviable adipose graft in the recipient site.[11] Fat necrosis in the face usually presents with a subcutaneous nodule, especially in the junction of the lower eyelid and cheek. It may require direct excision or precise liposuction for removal depending on severity of those conditions.

REVISIONS AND SUBSEQUENT PROCEDURES

In the author's practice, facial fat grafting is usually performed once for most patients with satisfactory outcome. However, subsequent fat

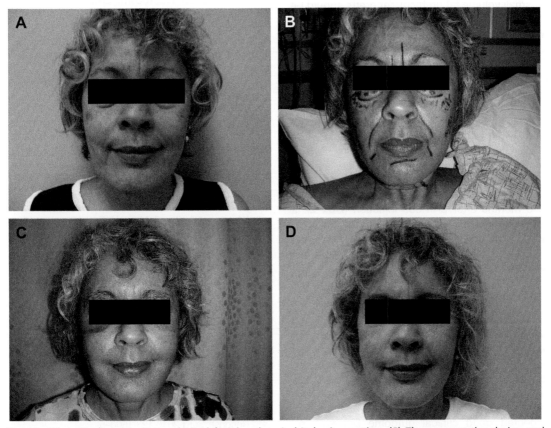

Fig. 16. (*A*) A 62-year-old woman desired facial and periorbital rejuvenation. (*B*) The preoperative design and plan for her facial and periorbital rejuvenation with fat grafting. She had a total of 25 cc fat grafts to her entire face (forehead: 2 cc; glabella: 2 cc; lower eyelid/cheek junction: 2 cc for each side; cheek: 2 cc for right side and 3 cc for left side; nasolabial fold: 3 cc for each side; mental crease: 2 cc; and perioral: 2 cc for each side). She also had bilateral upper and lower blepharoplasty, lateral canthopexy, and face and neck lifts. (*C*) The results at 6 weeks after her facial fat grafting and periorbital procedures and face and neck lift. (*D*) The results at 10-month follow-up.

grafting may be needed for some patients if additional fat grafting is necessary to improve clinical outcome. Occasionally some degree of asymmetry after fat grafting may be presented in an area of the face and gentle and precise liposuction should be performed to correct it.

CASE DEMONSTRATIONS

Case 1. See **Fig. 13**.
Case 2. See **Fig. 14**.
Case 3. See **Fig. 15**.
Case 4. See **Fig. 16**.

DISCUSSION

Much of the current scientific studies support this rationalized approach to facial fat grafting described in this article for small volume fat grafting.[23,24] Besides the proper selection of donor sites (ie, the lower abdomen or inner thigh for small volume fat grafting), fat grafts should be harvested with a less traumatic method such as syringe aspiration or lower suction pressure and then processed with proper centrifugation. Fat grafts should be placed in a small amount (no more than 0.1 cc or equivalent amount for large volume) each pass but with multiple passes in multiple tunnels, multiple tissue levels, and multiple directions. Anesthetic (or tumescent) solution with low lidocaine concentration should be chosen for infiltration of the donor site. Significant overcorrection should be avoided to minimize complications such as fat necrosis. The timing for subsequent injection may be about 3 to 6 months after previous injection (**Box 2**). It is also critical to inform the patient that a subsequent procedure may be necessary after the first fat grafting if the expected results have not been achieved.

SUMMARY

Improvement of fat grafting techniques can be accomplished with donor site selection, fat graft harvesting, processing, recipient site preparation, and placement. With the techniques and other important considerations described in this article, fat grafting can be performed in a more satisfactory fashion for facial rejuvenation with expected good clinical outcome but with no complications. Although a more rationalized approach to facial fat grafting is described by the author, future investigations may still be needed to provide more scientific evidences for what would be the best approach for facial rejuvenations.

Box 2
Summary of techniques and special considerations for facial fat grafting

Preferred donor sites	Lower abdomen or inner thigh
Anesthesia	Low concentration of lidocaine for infiltration
Fat graft harvesting	A less traumatic syringe technique
Fat graft processing	Centrifugation with a proper setting
Recipient site preparation	Injection of anesthetics for vasoconstriction. Percutaneous scar or adhesion release if needed.
Placement of fat grafts	Placed in a small amount (0.1 cc or equivalent amount) for each pass in the withdraw phase but with multiple passes in multiple tissue planes, multiple levels, and multiple directions
Overcorrection	Not recommended
Postoperative care	Proper immobilization of the grafted area. Swelling is always expected. Additional injection may be necessary
Timing for subsequent injection	3–6 mo after previous injection

REFERENCES

1. Coleman SR. Structural fat grafting: more than a permanent filler. Plast Reconstr Surg 2006;118: 108–120S.
2. Woodward J, Khan T, Martin J. Facial filler complications. Facial Plast Surg Clin North Am 2015;23: 447–58.
3. Coleman SR. Long-term survival of fat transplants: controlled demonstrations. Aesthetic Plast Surg 1995;19:421–5.
4. Coleman SR. Facial contouring with lipostructure. Clin Plast Surg 1997;24:347–67.
5. Del Vecchio D, Rohrich RJ. A classification of clinical fat grafting: different problems, different solutions. Plast Reconstr Surg 2012;130:511–22.
6. Keck M, Zeyda M, Gollinger K, et al. Local anesthetics have a major impact on viability of preadipocytes and their differentiation into adipocytes. Plast Reconstr Surg 2010;123:1500–5.
7. Carpaneda CA, Ribeiro MT. Percentage of graft viability versus injected volume in adipose autotransplants. Aesthetic Plast Surg 1994;18:17–9.
8. Sherman JE, Fanzio PM, White H, et al. Blindness and necrotizing fasciitis after liposuction and fat transfer. Plast Reconstr Surg 2010;126:1358–63.

9. Xie Y, Zheng DN, Li QF, et al. An integrated fat grafting technique for cosmetic facial contouring. J Plast Reconstr Aesthet Surg 2010;63:270–6.

10. Gutowski CA. Current applications and safety of autologous fat grafts: a report of the ASPS fat graft task force. Plast Reconstr Surg 2009;124:272–80.

11. Kanchwala SK, Glatt BS, Conant EF, et al. Autologous fat grafting to the reconstructed breast: the management of acquired contour deformities. Plast Reconstr Surg 2009;124:409–18.

12. Padoin AV, Braga-Silva J, Martins P, et al. Sources of processed lipoaspirate cells: influence of donor site on cell concentration. Plast Reconstr Surg 2008;122:614–8.

13. Geissler PJ, Davis K, Roostaeian J, et al. Improving fat transfer viability: the role of aging, body mass index, and harvest site. Plast Reconstr Surg 2014;134:227–32.

14. Yoshimura K, Suga H, Eto H. Adipose-derived stem/progenitor cells: roles in adipose tissue remodelling and potential use for soft tissue augmentation. Regen Med 2009;4:265–73.

15. Pu LLQ, Coleman SR, Cui X, et al. Autologous fat grafts harvested and refined by the coleman technique: a comparative study. Plast Reconstr Surg 2008;122:932–7.

16. Boscher MT, BeCkert BW, Puckett CL, et al. Analysis of lipocyte viability after liposuction. Plast Reconstr Surg 2002;109:761–5.

17. Pu LLQ, Cui X, Fink BF, et al. The viability of fatty tissues within adipose aspirates after conventional liposuction: a comprehensive study. Ann Plast Surg 2005;54:288–92.

18. Kurita M, Matsumoto D, Shigeura T, et al. Influences of centrifugation on cells and tissues in liposuction aspirates: optimized centrifugation for lipotransfer and cell isolation. Plast Reconstr Surg 2008;121:1033–41.

19. Pallua N, Pulsfort AK, Suschek C, et al. Content of the growth factors bFGF, IGF-1, VEGF, and PDGF-BB in freshly harvested lipoaspirate after centrifugation and incubation. Plast Reconstr Surg 2009;123:826–33.

20. Philips BJ, Grahovac TL, Valentin JE, et al. Prevelence of endogenous CD34$^+$ adipose stem cells predicts human fat graft rentention in a xenograft model. Plast Reconstr Surg 2013;132:845–58.

21. Kim IH, Yang JD, Lee DG, et al. Evaluation of centrifugation technique and effect of epinephrine on fat cell viability in autologous fat injection. Aesthet Surg J 2009;29:35–9.

22. Lee JH, Kirkham JC, McCormack MC, et al. The effect of pressure and shear on autologous fat grafting. Plast Reconstr Surg 2013;131:1125–36.

23. Pu LLQ. Towards more rationalized approach to autologous fat grafting. J Plast Reconstr Aesthet Surg 2012;65:413–9.

24. Lin JY, Wang CM, Pu LLQ. Can we standardize the techniques for fat grafting? Clin Plast Surg 2015;42:199–2018.

Fat Grafting for Facial Rejuvenation through Injectable Tissue Replacement and Regeneration
A Differential, Standardized, Anatomic Approach

Steven R. Cohen, MD[a,b], Hayley Womack, DO[a,c],*, Ali Ghanem, MD, PhD[d]

KEYWORDS

- Fat grafting • Anatomic fat grafting • Injectable tissue • Facial rejuvenation • Regenerative medicine
- ITR2

KEY POINTS

- Injectable Tissue Replacement and Regeneration (ITR[2]) is a standardized fat grafting technique, which anatomically addresses losses of facial volume, laxity, and sun damage of the skin.
- Anatomic components of volume loss are diagnosed through evaluation of facial surface topography and used to formulate unique, individualized treatment plans.
- Three sizes of fat grafts, millifat, microfat, and nanofat, are used to structurally replace losses in facial fat occurring at different depths and anatomic regions in the face.
- Regenerative effects of ITR[2] fat grafts often are augmented with regenerative cells obtained via mechanical fragmentation or through addition of stromal vascular fraction cell enrichment, platelet-rich plasma, and topical nanofat biocrème application.

 Video content accompanies this article at http://www.plasticsurgery.theclinics.com.

INTRODUCTION

Recent advances in understanding of facial aging have resulted in significant insights into facial soft tissue and bony volume loss. Lambros[1] documented photometric changes that showed that soft tissue of the face deflates with aging. Kahn

---

Disclosure Statement: Dr S.R. Cohen has stock options and royalties with Millennium Medical Technologies, Carlsbad, CA; has royalties with Tulip Medical; is a shareholder in the Mage Group, UK; and receives royalties on the Nanocube Device. He is an advisor for the Mage Group and Lipocube. He is an investigator for Allergan and Ampersand, Inc., and an investigator with Thermigen. The other listed authors have no competing financial disclosures or commercial associations. Ms H. Womack and Dr A. Ghanem have nothing to disclose.

[a] FACES+ Plastic Surgery, Skin and Laser Center, 4510 Executive Drive, #200, San Diego, CA 92121, USA; [b] Division of Plastic Surgery, University of California San Diego, 4510 Executive Drive, #200, San Diego, CA 9212, USA; [c] Division of Plastic Surgery, University of California San Diego, San Diego, CA, USA; [d] Blizard Institute, Barts and The London School of Medicine and Dentistry, Queen Mary University of London, 4 Newark Street, London E1 2AT, UK
* Corresponding author. 315 Goldenrod Avenue, Corona Del Mar, CA 92625.
E-mail address: hayleywomack222@gmail.com

Clin Plastic Surg 47 (2020) 31–41
https://doi.org/10.1016/j.cps.2019.08.005

and Shaw[2] and Mendelson and Wong[3] documented how the facial skeleton loses broad surface areas of bone without corresponding shrinkage of the soft tissue envelope. Rohrich and Pessa[4] clarified the anatomy of the superficial and deep fat compartments and recommended that fat be injected into specific deep fat compartments in the face because fat lies both above and below the facial musculature and ligaments. From the authors' own cadaver observations, fat is more tightly clustered in the superficial compartments above the muscles and larger and more loosely organized in the deep compartments below the facial musculature.

Advances in genetics have provided a basis for measuring early interventions that have the potential to slow aging of cells, and the finding of stem cells and regenerative cells in fat introduced the possibility of regenerating aging tissues, which was shown by Rigotti et. al[5–7] and supported by recent work by Cohen[8] and others.[9,10] There are almost no other therapies in aesthetics other than fat grafting, stromal vascular fraction (SVF)-enriched fat grafting, nanofat grafting, platelet-rich plasma (PRP), and growth factors, that have demonstrated neoangiogenesis and trophic effects to some degree in virtually all subjects.[7,11]

When patients come in for a facial aging consultation, they are evaluated at that particular moment in time. Yet, aging is an evolution of interdependent processes taking place over a lifetime. Growth dominates human development during the first 2 decades of life followed by a continual and gradual decay of tissues until death. The anatomic and histologic changes due to aging are seen individually in the skin, fat compartments, and underlying bone as well as dynamically in the interdependent relationships between them.[12] Facial aging can be anatomically and visually modeled from analysis of the topography of the face. The concept of injectable tissue replacement and regeneration (ITR[2]) attempts to answer a fundamental question: Can a dynamic model be used to determine the specific losses in facial fat compartments and bone and replace and/or regenerate these tissues in a way that reduces and to some extent reverses the facial aging process?

The ITR[2] procedure is a new, standardized method of differential fat grafting, which

1. Diagnoses the anatomic components of volume loss by evaluating the surface topography of the face
2. Addresses specific anatomic losses of different tissues, including skin, facial fat in the deep and superficial compartments, and bone

3. Replaces these anatomic losses of fat with 2 to 3 different sizes of autogenous fat grafts optimized in size for structural replacement for areas of bone and deep fat compartment losses, superficial fat compartment replacement, and dermal and epithelial replacement and/or regeneration

Regenerative effects of fat grafts may be augmented with regenerative cells obtained via mechanical fragmentation. For example, ITR[2] nanofat is primarily a matrix-rich product that is processed through microcutting of the aspirated adipose tissue using the Nanocube (Lipocube, London, United Kingdom) and contains matrix, adipocyte-derived stem cells, SVF cells and growth factors, PRP, and/or mechanically dissociated SVF.[13–16] This combination of anatomic fat replacement is supplemented with a menu of regenerative ingredients can be tailored to patient-specific needs.

PREOPERATIVE EVALUATION AND MARKINGS

The patient is marked with a white makeup pen while sitting in the upright position (Video 1). Scalp hair quality and/or loss are noted to determine if a restorative treatment a regenerative approach might be beneficial. The epidermal, dermal, and subcutaneous tissue thickness and the degree of bone recession in the glabella and along the supraorbital rims are noted in analyzing the upper third of the face. The degree of photodamage is noted. Deeper rhytids are noted for possible sharp-needle intradermal fat grafting (SNIF) technique.[17] Temporal depression is associated with deep fat loss, whereas increased show of the temporal veins is associated with superficial fat loss. Often both are present. The upper and lower eyelids and periorbital region are inspected. Loss of fullness of the lateral brow, loss of convexity of the skin caudal to the eyebrow, and supratarsal fold depth are noted. In the inferior orbit, the rim is evaluated as is the prominence of the intraorbital fat.

The tear trough and lid cheek junction are evaluated. The position of the globe is noted from the vertex view to determine the degree of proptosis. The lid to pupil position is noted and the degree of senile enophthalmos is evaluated. In the middle third, the zygomatic arch and body are outlined in white. The superior arch corresponds with the inferior temporal region. The deep lateral and medial suborbicularis occuli fat (SOOF) are noted as is the deep medial fat compartment of the cheek. The degree of buccal hollowing is evaluated. The nose is assessed for any aesthetic deformity and/or aging and the degree of pyriform recession is noted. The lips are evaluated along with the peri-oral tissues and degree of thinning and rhytids. In the lower third, the marionette basin is evaluated as the chin and labiomental fold. Chin texture may be improved with nanofat microneedling and fractional laser with topical delivery of nanofat biocrème. The prejowl area just lateral to the mandibular retaining ligaments, if scalloped, is addressed as is the inferior border of the mandible and the gonial angle. Chin projection is evaluated, and the neck is inspected for degree of subcutaneous loss, deep and fine rhytids and severity of sun damage.

SURGICAL PROCEDURES
Preoperative Preparation and Anesthesia

Patients are given oral prophylactic antibiotics 1 day before the procedure, if planned under local anesthesia, or intravenously before the procedure. Patients are given their choice of anesthesia, but for ITR[2], local or intravenous anesthesia and tumescent lipoharvest are used unless the patient is having other facial procedures. Patients are offered the possibility of undergoing a fixed focused ultrasound treatment, a week to a couple days before the procedure, for its potential release of endogenous angiogenic growth factors to prepare the recipient facial tissues.[18]

Adipose Tissue Harvest

If only fat grafting is being performed, the surgery itself takes approximately 45 minutes to an hour (see Video 1). Fat is harvested from any area of excess subcutaneous fat and/or areas of patient preference if sufficient fat is available. The patient is prepped and draped under sterile conditions. Harvest begins with a 14G needle puncture followed by infiltration of tumescent fluid (500 mL of Ringer lactate with 25 mg lidocaine and 1 vial of epinephrine [1:1000]). A 12-holed cannula, with openings measuring 2.5 mm in diameter (Marina Medical, Davie, Florida), is inserted into a slightly dilated 14G needle hole. Using a 60-mL syringe with a lock, fat is aspirated. Generally, 120 mL of fat is removed. These punctures are often allowed to close by secondary intention or by Dermabond (Ethicon, Bridgewater, New Jersey, US) wound adhesive.

Fat Processing

Once the fat is removed, the tumescent fluid is decanted, and the fat is rinsed with Ringer lactate to reduce blood contamination. Based on new research on fat preparation and degree of engraftment, filtration systems, such as Puregraft (Solana Beach, California), and centrifugation are probably not necessary and add to the cost.[19,20] Simple washing, gravity separation, and decantation to remove the tumescent solution are necessary to process the fat. When cleaning is complete, a portion of millifat is set to the side to replenish deep fat compartment loss and facial bone recession. The remaining fat is transferred into 20-mL syringes and processed into microfat and nanofat using the Nanocube kit, which has a total of 4 ports whose functions are to resize fat using a special cutting technique (see Video 1). Other systems that can process the various sizes of fat grafts can be used.

Delivery Techniques

According to the topographic assessment, fat grafts are assigned to anatomic locations in the face according to their parcel sizes of millifat (2–2.5 mm), microfat (1 mm), and nanofat (500 μm and less) (see Video 1). Placement starts with the deep compartments of the face and progresses superficially, using millifat first, then microfat, and ending with nanofat.

Up to 12 puncture sites are made with an 18G needle and are reused whenever possible in delivering the 3 sizes of fat grafts, shown in **Fig. 1**. Safe volume recommendations and sites for fat grafting are shown in **Fig. 2**.

MILLIFAT (2–2.5 MM PARCELS)
Middle Third/Temporal Region

Millifat is first placed through an 18G needle puncture in the nasolabial fold lateral and superior to the oral commissure, into the areas of bone recession in the pyriform region. The cannula is then directed cephalad to graft the deep medial fat compartment and the medial then lateral SOOF. The deep temporal region is grafted along with the preperiosteal lateral supraorbital brow. The upper and lower hemilip are injected with millifat at the commissure.

Upper Third

The glabella, medial supraorbital rims, and nasal radix are injected through a needle puncture in the central glabella, approximately 1.5 cm to 2 cm above the nasofrontal junction. The nasal dorsum, tip, and columella are then grafted through an entry point between the domes of the nasal tip.

ITR² PUNCTURE SITE CHRONOLOGY

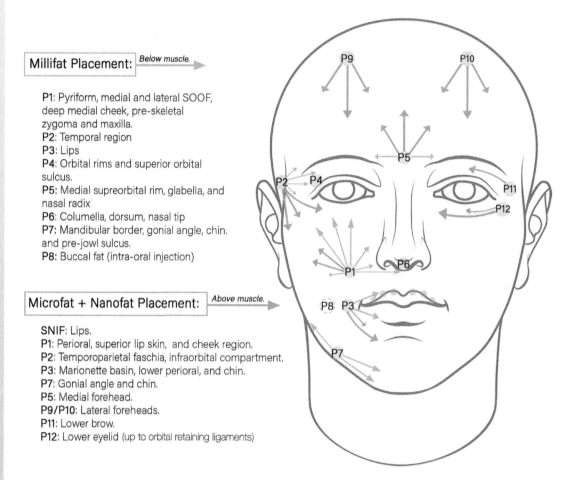

Millifat Placement: *Below muscle.*

P1: Pyriform, medial and lateral SOOF, deep medial cheek, pre-skeletal zygoma and maxilla.
P2: Temporal region
P3: Lips
P4: Orbital rims and superior orbital sulcus.
P5: Medial supreorbital rim, glabella, and nasal radix
P6: Columella, dorsum, nasal tip
P7: Mandibular border, gonial angle, chin, and pre-jowl sulcus.
P8: Buccal fat (intra-oral injection)

Microfat + Nanofat Placement: *Above muscle.*

SNIF: Lips.
P1: Perioral, superior lip skin, and cheek region.
P2: Temporoparietal faschia, infraorbital compartment.
P3: Marionette basin, lower perioral, and chin.
P7: Gonial angle and chin.
P5: Medial forehead.
P9/P10: Lateral foreheads.
P11: Lower brow.
P12: Lower eyelid (up to orbital retaining ligaments)

Please note: The injection sites displayed above should be utilizied on an as needed basis with regard to your patient's unique aging patterns. It is highly recommended that a topographical assessment is performed to apropriately plan where fat delivery will take place.

Fig. 1. Puncture site chronology and injection vectors used in ITR² fat grafting.

Lower Third

Attention is directed to the chin, mandibular border, and gonial angle. Modest retrogenia can be improved with millifat grafting. The area just lateral to the mandibular ligament and along the mandibular border is grafted in the preskeletal level through the same puncture. Millifat is placed along the inferior mandibular border and into the gonial angle to define the jawline, camouflage mild jowls, or lower an obtuse mandibular angle (see **Fig. 1**, puncture site "7" [P7]).

If the buccal fat compartment shows volume loss, it is injected using an intraoral approach (see **Fig. 1**, puncture site "8" [P8]). The patient is given intravenous clindamycin, and the intraoral mucosa just below Stensen duct is prepped with betadine and then punctured with an 18G needle. It is important to place only small amounts of fat into the deep buccal compartment and reinspect the area frequently to determine if the proper amount is injected. It is important not to overfill this lowlight area.

MICROFAT (1-MM PARCELS)
Middle Third and Temporal Regions

For the perioral skin, microfat is grafted superficially above the muscle from the nasolabial needle incision for the upper lip and the oral

ITR²

RECOMMENDED SAFE VOLUMES OF FAT PER SIDE

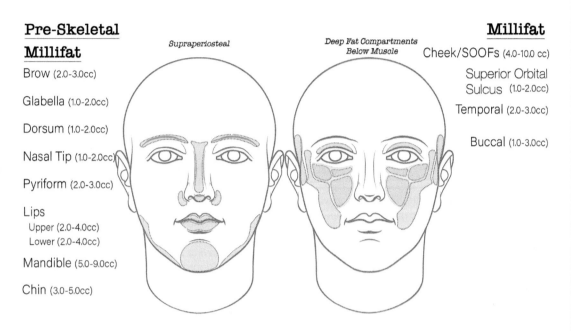

Pre-Skeletal Millifat

Supraperiosteal

Brow (2.0-3.0cc)

Glabella (1.0-2.0cc)

Dorsum (1.0-2.0cc)

Nasal Tip (1.0-2.0cc)

Pyriform (2.0-3.0cc)

Lips
Upper (2.0-4.0cc)
Lower (2.0-4.0cc)

Mandible (5.0-9.0cc)

Chin (3.0-5.0cc)

Deep Fat Compartments Below Muscle

Millifat

Cheek/SOOFs (4.0-10.0 cc)

Superior Orbital Sulcus (1.0-2.0cc)

Temporal (2.0-3.0cc)

Buccal (1.0-3.0cc)

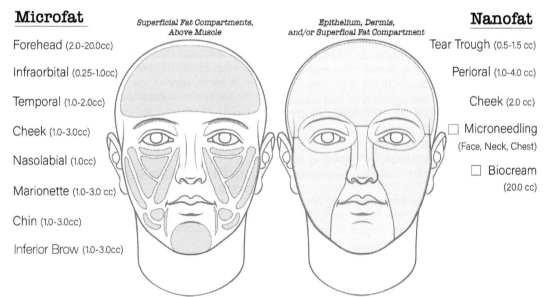

Microfat

Superficial Fat Compartments, Above Muscle

Forehead (2.0-20.0cc)

Infraorbital (0.25-1.0cc)

Temporal (1.0-2.0cc)

Cheek (1.0-3.0cc)

Nasolabial (1.0cc)

Marionette (1.0-3.0 cc)

Chin (1.0-3.0cc)

Inferior Brow (1.0-3.0cc)

Epithelium, Dermis, and/or Superficial Fat Compartment

Nanofat

Tear Trough (0.5-1.5 cc)

Perioral (1.0-4.0 cc)

Cheek (2.0 cc)

☐ Microneedling
(Face, Neck, Chest)

☐ Biocream
(20.0 cc)

Fig. 2. The recommended safe volume ranges with corresponding anatomic fat grafting locations.

commissure incision for the marionette basin and perioral tissue. The SNIF technique is used for the philtral columns (cupid's bow) and rhytids perpendicular to the white roll of the upper and lower lips.

The superficial temporal fat compartment is grafted with microfat using the same temporal puncture site as the deep temporal compartment (see **Fig. 1**, puncture site "2" [P2]).

Upper Third

For the forehead, the glabellar needle puncture site is used to inject superiorly and laterally into the medial brows (see **Fig. 1**, puncture site "5" [P5]). Two more needle incisions are then placed at the hairline on either side at the midpupillary line to graft the corresponding central, inferior, and lateral forehead subcutaneous (superficial) fat compartment.

The incision for the upper lid sulcus and lower brow fat pad is located on the lateral superior orbital rim approximately 3 mm inferior to the tail of the eyebrow. For the lower eyelid, 2 access points are used: the tear trough point (see **Fig. 1**, puncture site "11" [P11]) and a second point just lateral to the nasojugal groove (see **Fig. 1**, puncture site "12" [P12]). Microfat placement is in the supraperiosteal, preseptal space.

Lower Third

The subcutaneous fat of the chin and jawline, including the lateral superior gonial angle as well as the submental crease, are grafted with microfat to restore a uniform silhouette of the lower face (see **Fig. 1**, puncture site "7" [P7]).

NANOFAT (500-μM PARCELS)

Nanofat is placed using either the SNIF approach, topically with microneedling or with a topical biocrème. Until 2017, the authors prepared nanofat in the gradual emulsification technique originally described.[13] Since 2018, however, ITR[2] nanofat has been prepared using the Nancube. The advantage of the latter processing method is a matrix-rich product with less-traumatized regenerative cells.[21] When delivered through an SNIF technique for dermal rhytids, this cellularly optimized nanofat is injected intradermally using a 25G cannula attached to a finger-activated grafting device, 3-mL Celbrush (Cytori, San Diego, California), or an automatic grafting device, Lipopen (Juvaplus, Neuchâtel, Switzerland).

Finally, nanofat is delivered with a mechanical microneedling device into the face, neck, and décolletage. A 5-mL to 20-mL aliquot of nanofat is kept to combine with a transdermal liposomal carrier to form a topical nanofat biocrème (neo-U [Aries Biomedical, San Diego]).

POSTOPERATIVE CARE

Postoperative care consists of analgesia, nonsteroidal anti-inflammatory medications, and arnica for bruising. Direct application of ice is not permitted. Excessive swelling is treated as needed with a tapering oral steroid regimen. In patients undergoing facelift surgery or laser resurfacing, preoperative skin care is maintained with products containing matrikine (tripeptides and hexapeptides) ingredients

exhibiting biologic functions, which modulate extracellular matrix repair and neocollagenases (Alastin Skincare, Carlsbad, California).[22] In patients with a history of herpes simplex, perioperative prophylactic antivirals treatment is prescribed.

Patients can expect some bruising and swelling, with the lips swollen for approximately 5 days to 10 days. Patients can expect facial swelling and mild ecchymosis, which generally dissipate by day 3 to day 5, with 15% of patients taking longer, even a few weeks.

EXPECTED OUTCOME AND MANAGEMENT OF COMPLICATIONS

Patients having nanofat microneedling and/or nanofat biocrème (neo-U) in conjunction with fractional lasers of different wavelengths have experienced significant improvement in aesthetic outcomes with faster healing compared with historical controls that were not treated with nanofat. In patients having facelifts with ITR[2], facial volume improves by approximately 45% at a month, drops to approximately 25% to 30% from 7 months to 12 months, and then improves to 74% at 18 months to 24 months.[19] This finding suggests that there may be a reversal of tissue decay using ITR[2] in conjunction with facelift surgery.

Complications from ITR[2] have been rare and only related to excessive fat grafts in the lower eyelids. Although rare, transconjunctival or transcutaneous lower blepharoplasty with removal of fat has taken care of the problem. The authors no longer use microfat above the orbital retaining ligament, only matrix-rich nanofat. Since adopting ITR[2], the authors have not experienced any overgrowth with patient weight gain.

MAINTENANCE AND SUBSEQUENT PROCEDURES

Additional procedures are recommended based on a patient's physical findings and individual aging patterns.

CASE DEMONSTRATIONS
Patient 1

A 39-year-old woman demonstrates 6 years of aging (**Fig. 3**A, B). In **Fig. 3**C, she is shown 6 months post-ITR[2] and 2 years after ITR[2] (**Fig. 3**D). A total of 34 mL of fat was placed to the temporal, brows, cheeks, tear trough, nose, nasolabial folds, lips, and marionette lines. Note the gradual and subtle changes that occur with aging, the replacement of fat losses in the deep and superficial fat compartments, and her appearance after 8 years of aging.

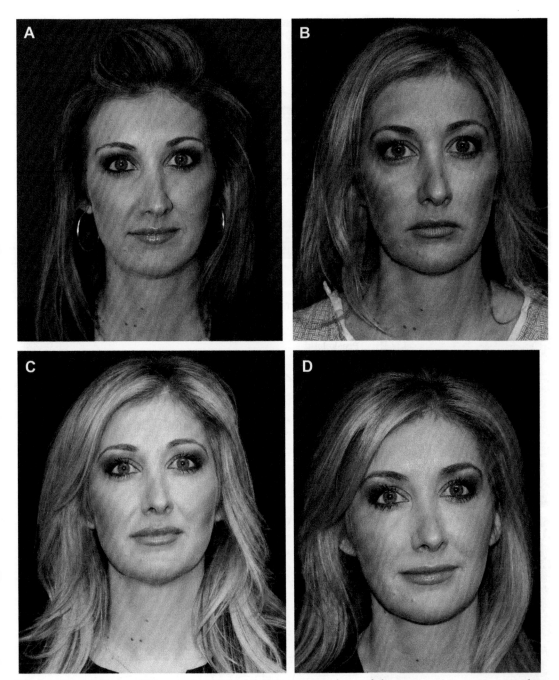

Fig. 3. Patient 1. Photo of 33-year old patient (*A*); Preoperative photo of the same patient at 39 years of age, demonstrating 6 years of natural aging (*B*); 6 months post-ITR2 (*C*); 2 years post-ITR2 (*D*). [Fig A–C (*From* Cohen SR, Womack H. Injectable tissue replacement and regeneration: anatomic fat grafting to restore decayed facial tissues. Plast Reconstr Surg Glob Open. 2019;7(8):e2293; with permission.)]

Patient 2

A 63-year-old woman is shown preoperatively, who presented with moderately severe skin laxity and volume loss (**Fig. 4**A). The purple overlays show the topographic planning and placement of millifat grafts (**Fig. 4**B). The green overlays show the topographic planning and placement of micro-fat grafts (**Fig. 4**C). The blue overlays show the topographic planning and placement of nanofat (**Fig. 4**D). The patient's face data sheet with the volumes of fat injected (**Fig. 4**E). Finally, the patient is shown 1 year postoperatively after being treated with upper and lower blepharoplasties, a high

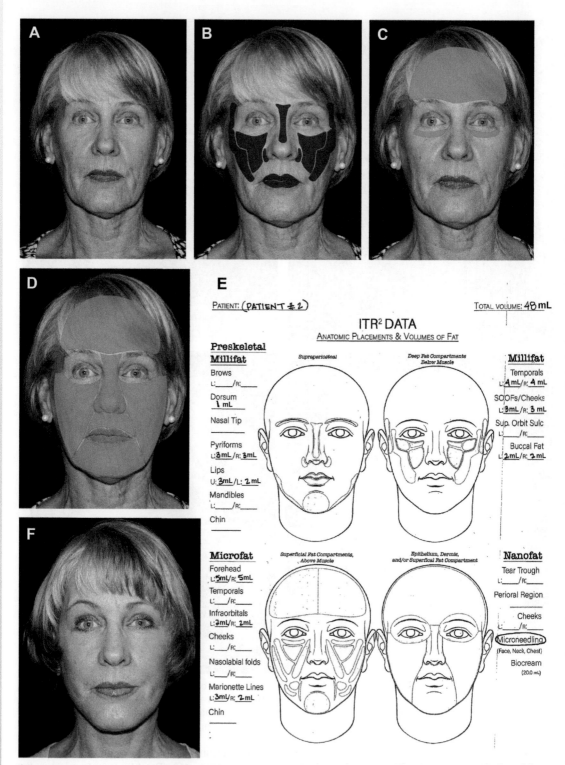

Fig. 4. Patient 2. A preoperative 63-year-old woman who presented with moderately severe skin laxity and volume loss (*A*). Topographic planning and placement of millifat grafts (*purple* [*B*]), microfat grafts (*green* [*C*]), and nanofat (*blue* [*D*]). Patient's face data sheet with the volumes of fat injected (*E*); 1 year postoperatively after being treated with upper and lower blepharoplasties, a high SMAS face and neck lift, and ITR² fat grafting, including the deep buccal fat compartment via a transoral approach (*F*).

superficial musculoaponeurotic system (SMAS) face and neck lift, and ITR^2 fat grafting, including the deep buccal fat compartment via a transoral approach (**Fig. 4**F).

Patient 3

Shown preoperatively, a 28-year-old man who was bothered by his lower eyelid hollowing and desired a regenerative approach (**Fig. 5**A). Shown again 6 months postoperatively after a total of 30 mL of millifat, microfat, and nanofat was used along with microneedling of the nanofat and postoperative nanofat biocrème (**Fig. 5**B).

Patient 4

Shown preoperatively, a 52-year-old woman who presented with concerns of periorbital aging and loss of facial volume (**Fig. 6**A). Patient is shown 1 year postoperatively after a total of 58.5 mL of fat was placed to the forehead, temporal regions, periorbital, perioral, midface, pyriform, and gonial angles (**Fig. 6**B). The patient also underwent skin-only upper blepharoplasty and pinch lower blepharoplasty. Note the improvement in globe position from the intraorbital fat grafting.

DISCUSSION

Currently, most surgeons and dermatologists inject fat aesthetically as if a filler, but fat is anatomically distributed in precise compartments of the face and should be placed in an anatomically correct fashion to avoid poor aesthetic results that can occur with weight gain. Because there is no fat present in the subcutaneous plane of the eyelid, nanofat is used exclusively to regenerate tissue because there is no structural requirement. Using an anatomic and regenerative approach seems to have 2 important benefits: (1) it addresses the actual anatomic changes that occur with aging, rather than simply using fat as a natural aesthetic filler, and (2) neoangiogenesis improves tissue health, possibly delaying atrophy of rete pegs and functional matrix, thus reducing the rate of laxity development and bone loss.

ITR^2 is an umbrella concept that incorporates knowledge of anatomic and histologic findings of facial aging with the ability to diagnose the areas of anatomic changes from the skin's surface to the bone. Although this approach may seem at first complex, it is simple, standardized, and routine to perform. Much as high-definition techniques during liposuction are predicated on an artistic understanding of anatomy, likewise, ITR^2 is based on being able to observe the anatomic changes of facial aging in different fat compartments, skin, and bone. Treatment is directed at all tissues that have decayed from epithelium to bone, using 2 sizes of fat grafts to address structural changes, superficial fat losses and skin thinning. Treatment using ITR^2 can be combined with other procedures on the eyelids and face. New ideas, such as

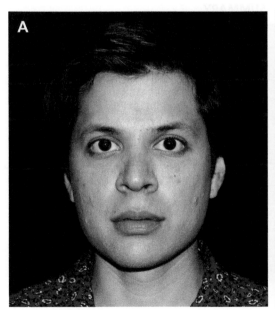
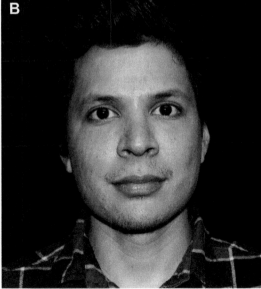

Fig. 5. Patient 3. A preoperative 28-year-old man who was bothered by his lower eyelid hollowing and desired a regenerative approach (*A*); 6 months postoperatively after a total of 30 mL of millifat, microfat, and nanofat was used along with microneedling of the nanofat and postoperative nanofat biocrème (*B*).

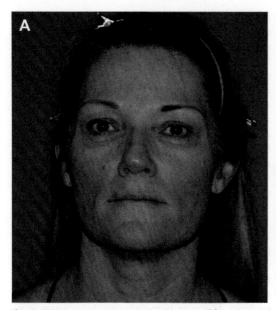 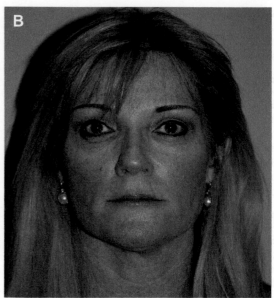

Fig. 6. Patient 4. A preoperative 52-year-old woman who presented with concerns of periorbital aging and loss of facial volume (*A*); 1 year postoperatively after a total of 58.5 mL of fat was placed to the forehead, temporal regions, periorbital, perioral, midface, pyriform, and gonial angles (*B*). (*From* Cohen SR, Womack H. Injectable tissue replacement and regeneration: anatomic fat grafting to restore decayed facial tissues. Plast Reconstr Surg Glob Open. 2019;7(8):e2293; with permission.)

injectable cartilage gel and injectable decellularized bone, are actively being explored.

It is possible to model the facial tissues as they progress from the period of growth and development to decay. The authors' concept involves stimulating the tissue with PRP and/or cellularly optimized nanofat at the earliest signs of decay to prevent the rapidity of these changes. Sun damage is treated with skin care and energy-based devices and lasers as needed. Skin care products with matrikine ingredients are used to clear the extracellular matrix of debris.[22] Aesthetic products, such as fillers, are used for beauty enhancement but have little to no effect on tissue health. Patients requiring more than one filler are excellent candidates for their first ITR[2] treatment of facial volume loss.

Studies are under way to determine the longevity of this approach, but the authors expect large standard deviations because they are now using the patient's own materials; therefore, variable results can be expected, that is, patients who age more rapidly or prematurely will benefit from different combinations of regenerative approaches, so some may require more treatments that others. New innovations, such as nanofat biocrème, nanofat microneedling, treatment of nasal aging with fat grafting and/or cartilage gel injections, buccal fat pad fat grafting, chin and jaw augmentation with decellularized allogeneic

bone, and intraorbital fat grafting to correct senile enophthalmos, are presented as new concepts under the umbrella of ITR[2] and may play important roles in the future of facial reconstruction and rejuvenation.

SUMMARY

ITR[2] presents a dynamic, anatomy-based approach to address patterns of facial aging, which occurs in specific superficial and deep fat compartments in the face. In addition, the ITR[2] technique delivers 3 structurally optimized fat grafts to replace and regenerate anatomic losses in the skin and deep and superficial fat compartments. The sizes of the nanofat, microfat, and millifat grafts are based on the structural differences of fat in these different areas and also make sense from a safety perspective.

SUPPLEMENTARY DATA

Supplementary data related to this article can be found online at https://doi.org/10.1016/j.cps.2019.08.005.

REFERENCES

1. Lambros V. Observations on periorbital and midface aging. Plast Reconstr Surg 2007;120(5):1367–76 [discussion: 1377].

2. Kahn DM, Shaw RB Jr. Aging of the bony orbit: a three-dimensional computed tomographic study. Aesthet Surg J 2008;28(3):258–64.

3. Mendelson B, Wong CH. Changes in the facial skeleton with aging: implications and clinical applications in facial rejuvenation. Aesthetic Plast Surg 2012;36(4):753–60.

4. Rohrich RJ, Pessa JE. The fat compartments of the face: anatomy and clinical implications for cosmetic surgery. Plast Reconstr Surg 2007;119(7):2219–27 [discussion: 2228].

5. Hannum G, Guinney J, Zhao L, et al. Genome-wide methylation profiles reveal quantitative views of human aging rates. Mol Cell 2012;49(2):359–97.

6. Zuk PA, Zhu M, Mizuno H, et al. Multilineage cells from human adipose tissue: implications for cell-based therapies. Tissue Eng 2001;7(2):211–28.

7. Rigotti G, Charles-de-Sá L, Gontijo-de-Amorim NF, et al. Expanded stem cells, stromal-vascular fraction, and platelet-rich plasma enriched fat: comparing results of different facial rejuvenation approaches in a clinical trial. Aesthet Surg J 2016; 36(3):261–70.

8. Cohen SR. Commentary on: expanded stem cells, stromal-vascular fraction, and platelet-rich plasma enriched fat: comparing results of different facial rejuvenation approaches in a clinical trial. Aesthet Surg J 2016;36(3):271–4.

9. Cytori therapeutics. Scleroderma treatment with celution processed adipose derived regenerative cells (STAR). In: ClinicalTrials.gov [Internet]. Bethesda (MD): National Library of Medicine (US). Available at: https://clinicaltrials.gov/ct2/show/NCT02396238. NLM Identifier: NCT02396238. Accessed January 1, 2018.

10. Cytori therapeutics. Celution prepared adipose derived regenerative cells in the treatment of osteoarthritis of the knee (ACT-OA knee). In: ClinicalTrials.gov [Internet]. Bethesda (MD): National Library of Medicine (US). Available at: https://clinicaltrials.gov/ct2/show/NCT02326961. NLM Identifier: NCT0232696. Accessed January 1, 2018.

11. Kamakura T, Kataoka J, Maeda K, et al. Platelet-rich plasma with basic fibroblast growth factor for treatment of wrinkles and depressed areas of the skin. Plast Reconstr Surg 2015;136(5):931–9.

12. Coleman SR, Grover R. The anatomy of the aging face: volume loss and changes in 3-dimensional topography. Aesthet Surg J 2006;26(1S):S4–9.

13. Tonnard P, Verpaele A, Peeters G, et al. Nanofat grafting: basic research and clinical applications. Plast Reconstr Surg 2013;132(4):1017–26.

14. Graziano A, Carinci F, Scolaro S, et al. Periodontal tissue generation using autologous dental ligament micro-grafts: case report with 6 months follow-up. Ann Oral Maxillofac Surg 2013;1:20.

15. Trovato L, Monti M, Del Fante C, et al. A new medical device rigeneracons allows to obtain viable micro-grafts from mechanical disaggregation of human tissues. J Cell Physiol 2015;230:2299–303.

16. Cervelli V, Gentile P, Scioli MG, et al. Application of platelet-rich plasma in plastic surgery: clinical and in vitro evaluation. Tissue Eng Part C Methods 2009;15:625.

17. Zeltzer A, Tonnard P, Verpaele A. Sharp-needle intradermal fat grafting (SNIF). Aesthet Surg J 2012; 32(5):554–61.

18. Reher P, Doan N, Bradnock B, et al. Effect of ultrasound on the production of IL-8, basic FGF and VEGF. Cytokine 1999;11(6):416–23.

19. Salinas HM, Broelsch GF, Fernandes JR, et al. Comparative analysis of processing methods in fat grafting. Plast Reconstr Surg 2014;134(4):675–83.

20. Cohen SR, Hewett S, Ross L, et al; Progressive improvement in midfacial volume 18 to 24 months after simultaneous fat grafting and facelift: an insight to fat graft remodeling, Aesthet Surg J. sjy279, https://doi.org/10.1093/asj/sjy279

21. Cohen SR, Tiryaki T, Womack HA, et al. Cellular Optimization of Nanofat: Comparison of Two Nanofat Processing Devices in terms of Cell Count and Viability. Aesthetic Surgery Journal Open Forum, in press.

22. Widgerow AD, Fabi SG, Palestine RF, et al. Extracellular matrix modulation: optimizing skin care and rejuvenation procedures. J Drugs Dermatol 2016; 15(4 suppl):s63–71.

Fat Grafting for Facial Rejuvenation in Asians

Zhibin Yang, MD, Ming Li, M.Med, Shengyang Jin, MD, Xinyu Zhang, MD, PhD, Xuefeng Han, MD, PhD, Facheng Li, MD, PhD*

KEYWORDS

• Fat grafting • Facial rejuvenation • Liposuction • Facial aging

KEY POINTS

- Preoperative communication with the patient, management of expectation, careful evaluation, and marking of the operation areas are critical to postoperative satisfaction.
- The infiltration of tumescent solution to recipient areas could decrease incidence of intraoperative hemorrhage, fat embolism and postoperative hematoma.
- Asians are characterized by depressed midface and wide facial contour, with fat grafting in the shape of a "T".
- Fat is mainly placed in the upper layer of periosteum and submuscular layer for structural support; a moderate amount of subcutaneous fat grafting forms a transition area with the surrounding tissue.
- The skin texture and color can be improved by microfat grafting for the subcutaneous and intradermal layers.

 Video content accompanies this article at http://www.plasticsurgery.theclinics.com.

INTRODUCTION

Fat grafting has been widely used in facial rejuvenation in recent years.[1,2] It can be applied to facial cosmetic alone or in combination with other facial lifting surgery.[3] With age, the skin relaxes with a decrease in elasticity, and sags caused by the relaxation of supporting ligaments, accompanied by the volume loss and redistribution of the deep and superficial fat compartment, as well as the absorption of the underlying bone,[4–8] all of which contribute to the senility of the facial morphology, such as facial hollowness and wrinkles.[9–13] In the past, the applications of facial skin and superficial musculoaponeurotic system fascia lifting surgeries were expected to achieve facial rejuvenation, but often did not produce satisfactory results. With the understanding of changes in facial fat pad of facial aging, and the studies of tissue regeneration of the adipose cell and adipose-derived stem cell, plastic surgeons gradually realized the importance of treating facial aging by restoring the volume of soft tissue and improving the texture of skin through fat grafting.

However, owing to the unpredictable absorption of the fat, plastic surgeons expect to obtain better results through overgrafting, which often result in complications such as fat necrosis, oil cysts, calcification, or overcorrection.[14] For the past 10 years, the authors have treated a large number of patients with facial rejuvenation by autologous fat grafting, acquiring satisfactory and long-lasting results without any severe complications. In this article, the authors introduce their preferred techniques of fat grafting for facial rejuvenation in Chinese patients.

Disclosure Statement: The authors have nothing to disclose.
Plastic Surgery Hospital (Institute), Chinese Academy of Medical Sciences, Peking Union Medical College, No. 33 Badachu Road, Shijingshan District, Beijing 100144, People's Republic of China
* Corresponding author.
E-mail address: drlfc@sina.com

Clin Plastic Surg 47 (2020) 43–51
https://doi.org/10.1016/j.cps.2019.08.003

PREOPERATIVE EVALUATION AND SPECIAL CONSIDERATIONS

It is crucial to communicate with the patient in detail to identify the patient's concerns and expectations. The patient should be made to understand the principles of fat grafting, therapeutic effects and complications to avoid unrealistic expectations and disappointment postoperatively.

The facial features and aesthetic standards of Asians are different from those of Caucasians. Asians have a low forehead, flattening midface, collapse of nose, and retraction of chin. For aesthetic appreciation, a full forehead and a raised nose and chin are considered to be a symbol of charm and glamour; the smoothness and softness of the curves on lateral face are more emphasized. The zygomatic arch and mandibular angle should not be protruding. Consequently, the sites for facial fat grafting are formed a region of a "T", aiming to create an inverted triangle on the face (**Fig. 1**).

In the youth (<35 years), fat grafting aims at the correction of the middle face congenital depression, while improving the outline of lateral face to form soft curves. For those greater than 35 years, the skin texture can be improved through the regeneration of microparticle fat grafted into the superficial layer of the face. Therefore, individualized design of the distribution and amount of graft

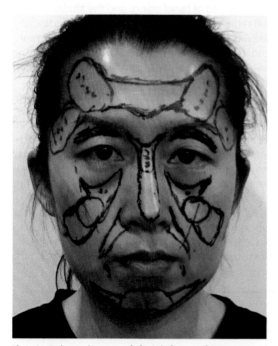

Fig. 1. T-shaped area of facial fat grafting: typical areas marked include forehead, temple, nose, tear trough, anterior cheek, nasolabial fold, and chin.

is performed according to gender, age, facial contour, skin texture, and degree of relaxation.

SURGICAL PROCEDURE
Donor Site Selection and Assessment

All fat deposits can be used as donor areas (Video 1). The purpose of surgery for some patients is not only to get facial rejuvenation, but also to improve body shape. Therefore, the patient's expectations can be used for reference in the selection of the donor areas. If only rejuvenation is sought, the authors usually prefer to select the abdomen or thigh as donor site for the following reasons. First, liposuction and facial lipofilling can be performed in the supine position without changing posture. Second, fat grafts can be obtained relatively easily in these areas. In addition, it has been reported that there are greater concentrations of adipose-derived stem cells in the lower abdomen and medial thigh.[15] It is a useful technique to assess the thickness of fat by skin grasping.

Fat Harvesting

The operation is generally carried out under intravenous or local anesthesia (if less fat is needed). The incisions of liposuction should be concealed. The incision is made 2 mm long with a No. 11 blade after anesthetized with 2.0 mL of 1% lidocaine and 1:100,000 epinephrine. A 2.0-mm diameter 9-hole cannula is used for infiltration anesthesia (**Fig. 2**A), and tumescent solution (490 mL normal saline, 10 mL 2% lidocaine, and 1 mL 1:1000 epinephrine) is infiltrated into the deep and superficial layers of the subcutaneous fatty tissue as the cannula moves forward and backward. In this way, the tumescent solution can penetrate uniformly and the fibrous connective tissue can be loosened, which is helpful in the subsequent liposuction. We adopt the tumescent technique for liposuction and the ratio of tumescent solution to fat harvested is 3:1, waiting for at least 15 minutes before beginning liposuction to attain adequate anesthesia and hemostasis.

Lipoaspirate is harvested through the same incisions previously made for infiltration of tumescent solution. There are 2 kinds of liposuction cannulas with the same diameter of 2.5 mm and 9 side holes, the hole sizes are 3.0 mm × 1.0 mm and 1.0 mm × 0.8 mm, and can be used to obtain fat parcels of different sizes (**Fig. 2**B). The macrofat is used to fill into the deep layer as structural support and volume augmentation, and the microfat is used precisely in the superficial layer to counteract the effects of skin aging.

The liposuction cannula connected to a 20-mL syringe is inserted into the incision and fat grafts

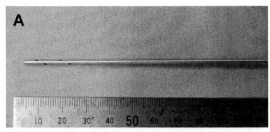

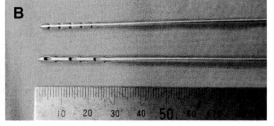

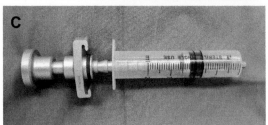

Fig. 2. A 2.0-mm diameter 9-hole anesthetic infiltration cannula (*A*). Two differences liposuction cannulas both are 25 cm in length and 2.5 mm in diameter with 6 side holes (*B*). A locking plunger is placed within a 20-mL syringe to harvest fat grafts (*C*).

is harvested with anterior and posterior movements (**Fig. 2**C). To ensure minimal mechanical trauma to the fat parcels, the plunger is pulled back gently at 2 to 4 mL to minimize negative pressure and maintained by locking. In general, the amount of fat harvested should be at least twice as much as anticipated to ensure that there is an adequate quantity for grafting.

Fat Processing

The authors are more inclined to adopt mesh/gauze for fat processing owing to its ability to remove more oily components and tumescent solution. It was reported that the fat obtained by the mesh/gauze technique contains more functional adipocytes and has a greater volume retention than that of the Coleman centrifugation technique.[16]

The obtained lipoaspirate is transferred into 60-mL syringes through a connector. After simple precipitation, the aqueous portion is discharged and an equal volume of normal saline is brought into the 60-mL syringe containing 25 mL of precipitated fat twice for rinsing to remove blood, cellular

debris, and any tumescent solution. After that, the fat is dumped on the metal filter with thick cotton pad below for 15 minutes to absorb any aqueous and oil components by capillary action. Meanwhile, the coarse fibrous tissues are manually removed to avoid cannula blockage. The purified fat is collected by 20-mL syringes and carefully transferred into 1-mm syringes through a connector. The fat should then be grafted immediately to minimize air exposure.

Preparation of the Recipient Site

An anesthetic block (usually including the supraorbital nerves, infraorbital nerves, and mental nerves) with 1% lidocaine and 1:200,000 epinephrine is particularly effective in reducing discomfort and pain while the patient is awake. The recipient areas are infiltrated with tumescent solution (0.04% lidocaine with 1:1000,000 epinephrine) using an 18-G pointed needle and a 3-hole cannula with a length of 7 cm and a diameter of 1.0 mm (**Fig. 3**A). We need about 50 mL of tumescent solution to infiltrate the entire face. The infiltration of tumescent solution can promote

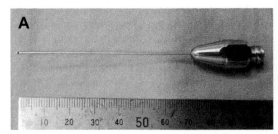

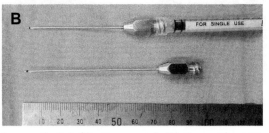

Fig. 3. A 7 cm in length, 1.0 mm in diameter and 3 side holes anesthetic infiltration cannula (*A*). Ranged from 5 to 7 cm in length and 1.2 mm in diameter blunt-tipped cannulas are used for fat grafting (*B*).

vasoconstriction to decrease the risk of a vascular embolism; the concomitant decrease in bleeding is beneficial to the survival of the fat because it decreases the inflammatory response. During the procedure, it should be emphasized that the areas just infiltrated should be pressed by the palm to mitigate the effect of swelling on the surgeon's judgment in the fat grafting process.

Fat Injection

The cannulas we used for fat grafting is blunt-tipped, 5 to 9 cm in length, and 1.0 or 1.2 mm in diameter (**Fig. 3**B).The key to fat grafting is to use a microdroplet technique with multiple layers from the periosteum to the subcutaneous layer. The fat is injected while the cannula is withdrawn, avoiding injection into the blood vessels. The end plunger of syringe should be held in the palm of the hand to control injection pressure and avoid overinjection.

Upper facial fat grafting

Entry points of fat injection for forehead are located at the edge of hairline and additional entry points can be made at the eyebrow tail (**Fig. 4**). It is essential to mark the projection of supraorbital vessels and supratrochlear vessels on the surface of supraorbital margin. The supraorbital vessels

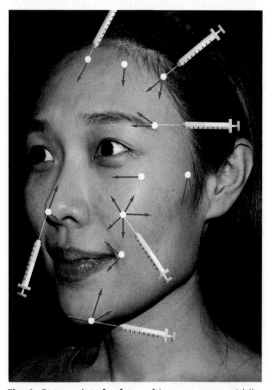

Fig. 4. Entry points for fat grafting on upper, middle, and lower face.

and nerves leave the supraorbital notch and run upward about 0.5 to 1.0 cm on the periosteum before entering into the frontal muscle.[17] The supratrochlear vessels and nerves that have a 1-cm distance to the medial orbit of the supraorbital notch pass through the orbital margin and then immediately enter into the superficial layer of frontal muscle. Therefore, within the range of the superior orbital margin (2 cm at the medial of pupil vertical line), the fat should be placed meticulously in the subcutaneous layer rather than periosteal layer. In contrast, in other parts of forehead the fat, as a structural support, is mainly placed on the periosteum to augment the lost volume resulting from deep fat atrophy. Small doses of fat should be dispersed subcutaneously, forming a smoother and more natural transition to the surrounding regions. Excessive placement of fat in subcutaneous layer can affect the expression of mimetic muscle. The forehead will take on a clear accumulation of fat, presenting balloon-like appearance. According to the inherent contour and depression of patient's forehead, the total amount of fat grafts ranges from 5 to 20 mL.

For injection into the temple, eyebrow arch, and upper eyelid, an entry site can be made at the eyebrow tail and another entry point as access to the temple is located at the junction of temporal line and hairline. There is an areola space between the superficial temporal fascia and the deep temporal fascia where more fat should be placed to enlarge the volume of temporal fossa. Although the superficial temporal artery, zygomatic orbital artery, and temporal branch of the facial nerve are distributed in the superficial temporal fascia, infusing fat into the areola space with a blunt-tipped cannula does not normally damage these blood vessels and nerves. However, the anterior part of the lower temporal compartment, that is, the region about 1 fingerbreadth above the zygomatic arch at the lateral orbital margin, has the sentinel vein and branches of the middle temporal vessels passing through, so particular attention should be paid to the manipulation in this area.[18] A proper amount of fat grafting should also be performed subcutaneously in the temporal region, avoiding overcorrection of the lateral orbital margin to increase the width of the face. The fat volume in the temporal region is between 3 and 15 mL on each side.

A blunt-tipped cannula that is 1.0 mm diameter can be used to fill the sunken upper eyelid. The operator or assistant should pull the eyebrows to the side of the head to maintain the tension of upper eyelid skin, so that the cannula has easy access to the area below the orbicularis oculi muscle through the entry point of the eyebrow tail for fat injection in this area. For each side, 0.5 to 2.0 mL of fat is needed. The subcutaneous layer should be avoided because injecting fat there can result in complications such as bloated upper eyelids, laborious eye opening, palpable oil cysts, and nodules.

Middle facial fat grafting

The site of anterior cheek serves as an entry point for middle facial fat transplants, where the fat can be easily placed in the inferior lower eyelid, medial and lateral cheeks, and nasolabial fold. An additional entry point may also be made at the suborbital lateral margin as a supplement, allowing access to the suborbital region and anterior cheek regions (see **Fig.4**).

For correction of the palpebral cheek sulcus and palpebral zygomatic sulcus deformity, first the larger fat parcels should be deposited in the periosteum and suborbicularis oris fat layers along the inferior orbital rim as structural support, and then the microfat parcels should be meticulously placed in the subcutaneous to avoid irregular nodules. When the cannula is closing to the lower orbital rim, the index finger of the nondominant hand should touch the inferior orbital rim to guide the cannula to inject the fat into the proper position and prevent the cannula from penetrating the eyelid conjunctiva and injuring the eyeball. A total of no more than 3 mL of fat is placed per side. Overcorrection in these areas is not recommended.

Fat grafting in the anterior cheek is critical to facial rejuvenation; it provides highlight projection. This injection can be undertaken in all layers, including deep, middle, and superficial, through the entry points of the anterior cheek and suborbital lateral margin.

To smooth out the nasolabial fold, fat should be placed in multiple layers in a fan-shaped manner, especially in the Ristow space of nasal alar basal region (Ristow B. Personal communication, 2001). The critical technique is infiltration of the areas around the folds rather than a linear placement that will aggravate the original creases. Avoid placing fat grafts in the superficial nasolabial fat pad, because the fat pad in this area is mainly displaced downward rather than reduced with age. On each side, 2 to 4 mL of fat is required.

For correction of the lateral cheek depression, the entry point is located at the leading edge of the sideburns. Fat should be placed on the surface of the masseter fascia and parotid gland, as well as subcutaneously, with special care to avoid injuring the deep important tissues. The volume placed varies from 5 to 15 mL in each cheek area.

Lower facial fat grafting

For fat grafting of the lower face, we select both sides of the mental edge as entry points, allowing the cannula to readily approach to the chin, bottom of the lips, and lateral of mandible. Additional entry points can be made as needed such as the lateral of oral commissure, which can be used for fat grafting to the upper and lower lips (see **Fig. 4**).

Fat can be placed in multiple levels of the chin. Aponeurosis tissue tightly attached to the

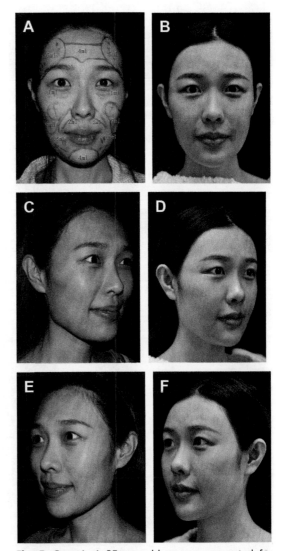

Fig. 5. Case 1. A 35-year-old woman presented for facial rejuvenation with fat grafting. Preoperatively, this patient demonstrated the temporal hollowness and sunken buccal region (A, C, E). Fat grafting was performed with a total of 39 mL in the forehead, temples, medial and lateral cheeks, inferior lower eyelids, nasolabial folds. One year after surgery showed removal of shadows on both sides of the face and a youthful appearance (B, D, F).

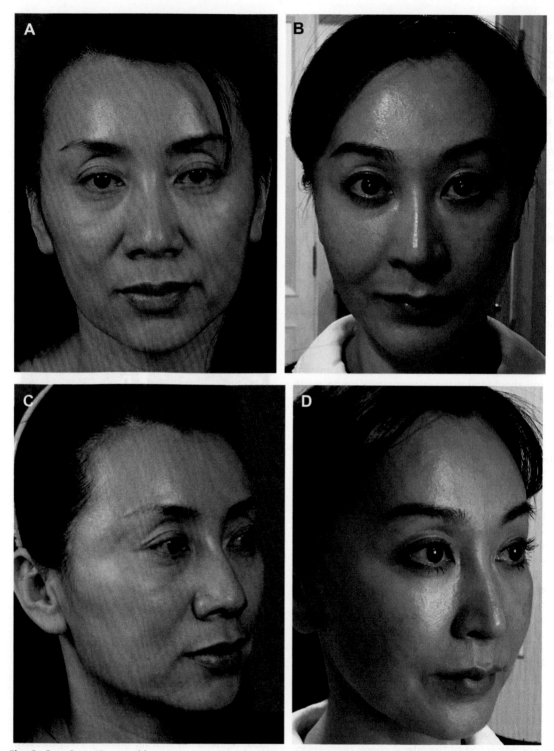

Fig. 6. Case 2. A 47-year-old woman presented for fat grafting to restore his forehead, temples, anterior and lateral cheeks, upper and lower eyelids, anterior and lateral cheeks, nasolabial folds and chin (before the operation in *A* and *C*; 1 year after the operation in *B* and *D*).

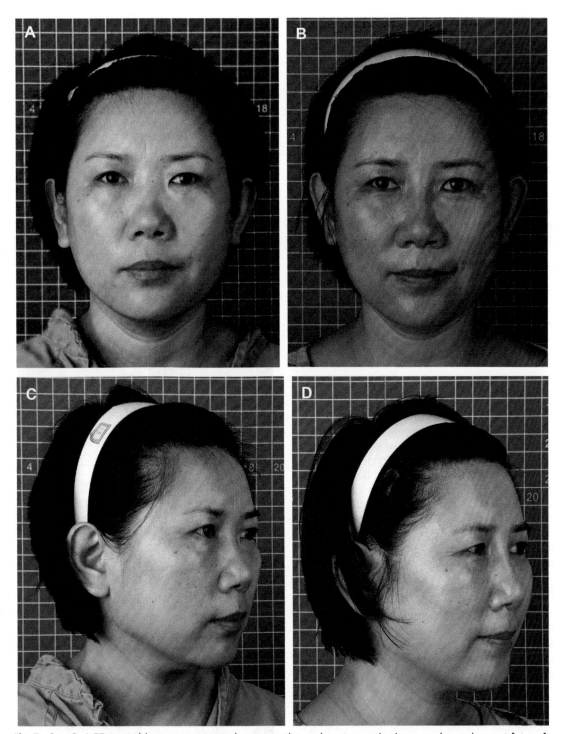

Fig. 7. Case 3. A 55-year-old woman presented preoperative and postoperative images who underwent fat grafting for augmentation rhinoplasty (before the operation in *A* and *C*; 1.5 years after the operation in *B* and *D*) .

periosteum can be stripped off with a blunt cannula, thus, expanding the space to facilitate fat survival. For patients with insufficient mental protrusion, the improvement of lower facial aesthetics is mainly to increase the chin horizontally rather than vertically. In other areas, fat grafting is needed are on both sides of the chin, where significant hollowing occurs with age.

For correction of the droop of mouth angle, volume restoration of atrophic fat by placing fat into the deep layers under orbicularis muscle can obtain satisfactory effect. The effacement of marionettes lines involves fat infiltration around the wrinkles in a crossed manner, similar to that of nasolabial fold. The aggravation of marionettes lines is not only caused by the atrophy of labio-mandibular fat pad, but also by the ptosis and hypertrophy of jowl fat.[12] Therefore, when the effect of fat grafting alone is not satisfactory, the authors' experience was to combine fat grafting with facial liposuction and facial lifting surgery to get better aesthetic results. The amount of fat grafted for the lower face is approximately 3 to 10 mL per side, depending on the individual needs.

POSTOPERATIVE CARE

Remove sutures after 5 days and forbid facial massage for 1 month. For liposuction of a large area, we recommend that the patient should wear an elastic garment for at least 6 weeks to pressurize the donor areas.

Expected Outcome and Management of Complications

Facial fat grafting is relatively safe with a high satisfaction rate and a relatively low complication rate in the hands of experienced surgeons. Complications include fat accumulation, asymmetry, hematoma, infection, cyst formation, fibrosis, calcification, and irregularity at the donor sites. Vascular embolism, although rare, can result in catastrophic consequences. The authors have been performing fat grafting for facial rejuvenation for many years and obtained favorable long-term results without severe complications.

REVISION OR SUBSEQUENT PROCEDURES

Approximately 40% of patients with inadequate facial correction achieved satisfactory outcomes after a secondary touch-up procedure. The interval between the operations should be at least 6 months.

CASE DEMONSTRATIONS

Photographs of 4 representative patients are illustrated in **Figs. 5–8**.

DISCUSSION

Fat grafting has been widely used in facial rejuvenation. However, clinical results vary greatly resulting from the multiple procedures involved and serious complications have been reported

from time to time. Fat harvesting was done by syringe with low pressure to minimize mechanical damage to the adipocytes. Then, the fat was rinsed by normal saline and processed by mesh/gauze technique for removal of the debris, oil, and inflammatory components. A small amount of tumescent solution was injected in the recipient sites for vasoconstriction and to make space for fat injection. Fat is mainly placed in the upper layer of periosteum and submuscular layer for structural support and correction of hollow areas. Meanwhile, facial wrinkles can be alleviated and a natural transition into the adjacent areas can be achieved by appropriate grafting in the superficial subcutaneous layer. Although inadequate correction is commonly seen, overcorrection is not recommended because it increases the incidence of complications. The graft gradually incorporated and inflammation subsided 6 months postoperatively. A second procedure can be performed for patients who did not achieve desired results. At

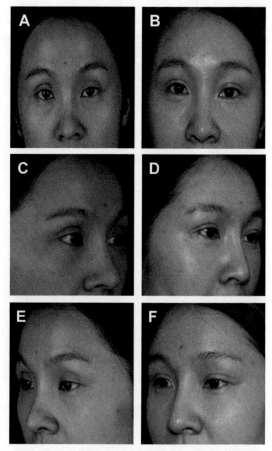

Fig. 8. Case 4. A 41-year-old woman presented for fat grafting to restore his forehead, temples, nose, anterior cheeks, upper and lower eyelids (before the operation in A, C, and E; 1 year after the operation in B, D, and F).

present, although we have made great progress on operative skills, the unpredictability of fat survival remains a problem. The authors expect further developments in basic experimental and clinical practices to achieve higher survival rates for the fat grafting. More accurate treatment can be performed with the aid of various methods, such as the 3-dimensional volume measurement.

SUMMARY

Fat grafting is a safe and effective measure for facial rejuvenation. It is of importance to understand comprehensively the mechanism and the role of volume loss in facial aging. Satisfactory results can be achieved if plastic surgeons are skilled in applying the strategies described in this article.

SUPPLEMENTARY DATA

Supplementary data to this article can be found online at https://doi.org/10.1016/j.cps.2019.08.003.

REFERENCES

1. Coleman SR. Structural fat grafting: more than a permanent filler. Plast Reconstr Surg 2006;118(3): 108S–20S.
2. Marten TJ, Elyassnia D. Fat grafting in facial rejuvenation. Clin Plast Surg 2015;42(2):219–52.
3. Rohrich RJ, Afrooz PN. Finesse in face lifting: the role of facial fat compartment augmentation in facial rejuvenation. Plast Reconstr Surg 2019;143(1): 98–101.
4. Furas DW. The retaining ligaments of the cheek. Plast Reconstr Surg 1989;83(1):11–6.
5. Pessa JE, Chen Y. Curve analysis of the aging orbital aperture. Plast Reconstr Surg 2002;109(2):751–5.
6. Shaw RB Jr, Kahn DM. Aging of the midface bony elements: a three-dimensional computed tomographic study. Plast Reconstr Surg 2007;119(2): 675–81 [discussion: 682–3].
7. Mendelson B, Wong CH. Changes in the facial skeleton with aging: implications and clinical applications in facial rejuvenation. Aesthetic Plast Surg 2012;36(4):753–60.
8. Mendelson BC, Hartley W, Scott M, et al. Age-related changes of the orbit and midcheek and the implications for facial rejuvenation. Aesthetic Plast Surg 2017;31(5):419–23.
9. Rohrich RJ, Pessa JE. The fat compartments of the face: anatomy and clinical implications for cosmetic surgery. Plast Reconstr Surg 2007;119(7):2219–27 [discussion: 2228–31].
10. Donofrio LM. Fat distribution: a morphologic study of the aging face. Dermatol Surg 2000;26(12): 1107–12.
11. Gierloff M, Stöhring C, Buder T, et al. Aging changes of the midfacial fat compartments: a computed tomographic study. Plast Reconstr Surg 2012; 129(1):263–73.
12. Gierloff M, Stöhring C, Buder T, et al. The subcutaneous fat compartments in relation to aesthetically important facial folds and rhytides. J Plast Reconstr Aesthet Surg 2012;65(10):1292–7.
13. Wan D, Amirlak B, Giessler P, et al. The differing adipocyte morphologies of deep versus superficial midfacial fat compartments: a cadaveric study. Plast Reconstr Surg 2014;133(5):615e–22e.
14. Yoshimura K, Coleman SR. Complications of fat grafting: how they occur and how to find, avoid, and treat them. Clin Plast Surg 2015;42(3):383–8.
15. Geissler PJ, Davis K, Roostaeian J, et al. Improving fat transfer viability: the role of aging, body mass index, and harvest site. Plast Reconstr Surg 2014; 134(2):227–32.
16. Canizares O Jr, Thomson JE, Allen RJ Jr, et al. The effect of processing technique on fat graft survival. Plast Reconstr Surg 2017;140(5):933–43.
17. Seckel BR. Facial danger zones: avoiding nerve injury in facial plastic surgery. 2nd edition. St Louis (MO): Quality Medical Publishing Inc; 2010.
18. Huang RL, Xie Y, Wang W, et al. Anatomical study of temporal fat compartments and its clinical application for temporal fat grafting. Aesthet Surg J 2017; 37(8):855–62.

Fat Grafting for Facial Rejuvenation with Nanofat Grafts

Patrick Tonnard, MD, PhD[a],*, Alexis Verpaele, MD, PhD[a],
Marcelo Carvas, MD[b],[1]

KEYWORDS

- Nanofat • Needling • Rejuvenation • Stem cell • Regenerative • Antiaging

KEY POINTS

- Nanofat has no filling capacity. It is a highly concentrated solution of progenitor cells and has no viable adipocytes.
- The mechanical protocol for nanofat preparation is essential. It consists of a 2-step emulsification technique followed by filtration.
- Striking improvement on the skin quality is perceived 6 to 8 months after nanofat grafting. Association of hyaluronic acid, botulin toxin, and vitamin C provides shorter-term enhancement of the skin quality.
- Grafting can be performed by a nanofat intradermal injection or by a microneedling delivery system. Nanofat cream is used as an adjunct after the procedure to further maximize benefit and to moisturize the skin during initial healing.

 Video content accompanies this article at "http://www.plasticsurgery.theclinics.com".

INTRODUCTION

During the past 20 years, lipofilling has emerged as a fundamental component in a facial rejuvenation procedure (Video 1). Currently, facelifts and lipofilling can be almost considered inseparable: facelift techniques address the sagging process, whereas the lipofilling focuses on the deflation. First described in 2001,[1] adipose-derived stem cells (ADSCs) and their therapeutic potential may be the tool researchers and clinicians were looking for to address the third component of the aging process: the structural changes of the skin. For the past decade, these fat tissue cells have shown not only biocellular regenerative potential in vitro but also striking improvement of the quality of skin in clinical cases.[2–4] Adipose tissue is easily harvested by minimally invasive liposuction and a large number of mesenchymal stem cells are obtained in the lipoaspirate. The wide availability of adipose tissue combined with the straightforward mechanical protocol to process the fat into a highly concentrated solution of progenitor cells brings regenerative medicine into real-life clinical practice. In 2013, Tonnard and colleagues[2] described the procedure to produce so-called nanofat out of harvested microfat by a simple mechanical emulsification.

The mechanical protocol consists of emulsification of the harvested microfat, followed by

Disclosure Statement: Dr P. Tonnard and Dr A. Verpaele receive royalties from Tulip Medical, San Diego, CA, USA, for certain instruments. Dr M. Carvas has nothing to disclose.
[a] Coupure Centrum voor Plastische Chrirugie, Coupure Rechts 164, Ghent B-9000, Belgium; [b] Clinique Faria Lima, São Paulo, Brazil
[1] Present address: Coupure Rechts 164, Ghent B-9000, Belgium.
* Corresponding author.
E-mail address: patrick@coupurecentrum.be

Clin Plastic Surg 47 (2020) 53–62
https://doi.org/10.1016/j.cps.2019.08.006

filtering.[2] The result is a whitish liquid with no viable adipocytes but with a large number of good-quality mesenchymal stem cells. Although adipocytes represent 80% to 90% of the volume of the harvested fat, they only represent 25% of the cell count.[5] The remaining 75% is called the stromal vascular fraction (SVF). This contains a large amount of ADSCs, as well as endothelial cells, monocytes, macrophages, granulocytes, and lymphocytes.

The regenerative mechanism by which nanofat works is still not completely understood. Studies suggest that the multiple cell types in the SVF might work in combination to provide a microenvironment where numerous markers come together and trigger the regenerative capacity of the stem cell and of the tissue itself.[4] Recent research has shown that the mechanical shear stress imposed on the fat during preparation of nanofat generates an upregulation of signaling pathways to enhance multipotent and pluripotent stem cells' capacity to regenerate.[6] The results of these complex intercellular crosstalking reactions were reported to range from enhanced collagen deposition and skin elasticity to formation of new blood vessels, tissue remodeling, thickening of the dermis, and downregulation of melanogenic activity.[7–11] This wide range of regenerative properties brings nanofat grafting into focus for both cosmetic and reconstructive surgery.[12]

This article describes the techniques and the authors' experiences in nanofat grafting, as well as its potential new applications in regenerative medicine.

PREOPERATIVE EVALUATION AND SPECIAL CONSIDERATIONS

With the clinically perceived benefit of nanofat and its applications, the authors are presently offering it to all our patients in whom at least 1 of the following items is present:

1. Trophic skin changes associated with age and photodamage
   - Thin dermis
   - Fine wrinkles
   - Craquelé surface (ie, neck, décolleté, perioral)
   - Mucosal aging (ie, dry lips, genital)
2. Pigmentary conditions
   - Pigmentary changes (ie, face, hands)
   - Dark circles under the eye in cases of thin dermis associated with increased melanin pigment deposits
3. Scarring and atrophy
   - Scars
   - Radiodermatitis.

There are no specific contraindications of its use and only transient yellowish staining is sometimes seen in the first postoperative week, followed by a mild inflammation that can last up to 3 weeks.

Nanofat does not have filling capacity. Thus, the idea in nanofat grafting is injecting regenerative cells and extracellular elements to promote tissue regeneration and remodeling. Clinically, nanofat grafting can be done alone or in association with other rejuvenation procedures (ie, facelift and lipofilling). Indications for nanofat extend beyond facial rejuvenation procedures; areas such as the neck, décolleté, and hands can also benefit from its use. Overall improvement of the quality of the overlying skin can be perceived after 6 to 8 months. Reported changes range from improvement in elasticity, pigmentary conditions, texture, and fine wrinkles.[2,3,8,10–12] Its versatility, simplicity, and safety made nanofat an integral component of the authors' clinical practices.

SURGICAL PROCEDURE
Harvesting

After infiltration of modified Klein solution (1:1.000.000), microfat is harvested under full-force vacuum aspiration into a sterile canister. The use of a fine 2.4-mm cannula with 20 1-mm sharpened holes (Tulip Medical, San Diego, CA, USA) was associated with an increased rate of ADSCs in the microfat when compared with conventional harvested fat.[13,14] The lipoaspirate is then rinsed with saline or Ringer's lactate over a sterile nylon cloth with 0.5-mm perforations mounted on a sterile canister. After removal of fibrous remnants with a mosquito, the obtained microfat is transferred to 10-mL Luer-Lok syringes.

Nanofat Preparation by Intersyringe Shuffling

The mechanical protocol of nanofat preparation consists of a 2-step emulsification process followed by filtration. The first step is performed by vigorous shifting of the microfat from a full 10-mL syringe to an empty one through a 2.4-mm female-to-female Luer-Lok connector (Tulip Medical, San Diego, CA, USA). After 30 passes, the same process is repeated with a 1.2-mm female-to-female Luer lock connector for another 30 vigorous passes. This progressive emulsification process is important to guarantee that all adipocytes are destroyed. At the end of this emulsification process, a whitish discoloration of the fat is seen. The fat is now passed through a double 400-micron or 600-micron filter (disposable filter or permanent strainer cartridge) to remove connective tissue remnants (Tulip Medical, San Diego,

CA, USA). When nanofat needling is planned, for every 10 mL of nanofat obtained, 1 mL of hyaluronic acid (HA) filler (cost ± €80), 100 mg of vitamin C, and 50 units of botulin toxin (cost ± €60) are added and mixed together. Preparation of the nanofat cream consists of mixing equal volumes of cream and nanofat.

Preparation of Recipient Site

When performed under local anesthesia, nanofat injections and nanofat needling to the face are well-tolerated after facial nerve blocks using lidocaine 1% (supraorbital, supratrochlear, infraorbital, and mental nerves). For neck and décolleté treatment, topical anesthesia (lidocaine 5% cream applied for 40 minutes before procedure) is usually sufficient. Under general anesthesia, no extra infiltration or block is needed. Marking from the earlier microfat grafting is removed before the needling to avoid transcutaneous tattooing.

Combining Treatment Modalities

Clinically, improvement of the quality of skin after nanofat grafting can be perceived after a minimum of 6 to 8 months. In an attempt to provide a shorter term enhancement of skin quality, the authors used a novel delivery system and used microbotox, skin booster HA, and vitamin C in our clinical practices, with obvious immediate results.

Microneedling

The authors first described the method of delivering nanofat through intradermal injection using 27-gauge needles. Although this approach is very effective for small areas, such as upper lip and eyelids, addressing bigger areas is time-consuming and it may be difficult to deliver the nanofat emulsion evenly throughout the area. Full-face treatment, as well as neck and décolleté treatment, benefit from a different delivery method.

Verpaele and colleagues[15] recently described a novel method of nanofat delivery using a microneedling device (**Fig. 1**), the Hydra Needle 20 (Guangzhou Ekai Electronic Technology Co Ltd, Guangzhou, China). This method not only allows uniform delivery of nanofat in the created microchannels but also associates with the benefits of the microneedling itself. Microneedling is a well-established skin treatment that works by percutaneous collagen induction trough activation of a series of growth factors.[16] Combining the regenerative capacity of the nanofat with the additional stimulus of collagen production and scarless healing provided by the needling may work synergistically to optimize results.[12] The device contains 20 1.5-mm needles and is used by repetitive tapping

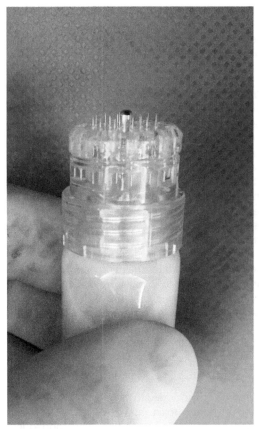

Fig. 1. Hydra Needle 20 (Guangzhou Ekai Electronic Technology Co Ltd, Guangzhou, China) microneedling device. The 8-mL vial has a pump-system that delivers microdroplets of nanofat after each tapping motion. The device's lid contains 20 1.5-mm needles.

motions to create the microchannels. The papillary dermis is reached as reflected by the punctuate bleeding obtained. The pump system in the needling device delivers the content of each bottle (up to 8 mL each) in thousands of tiny droplets of nanofat into the dermis. Needling is normally performed for 20 minutes, the time to empty the 8 mL vial.

Microbotox

The concept of microbotox was introduced by Wu[17,18] in 2001. Instead of acting in deep muscles, the idea of microbotox is to act on the quality of the skin itself. Through a very superficial and uniform technique of injection into the dermis, the botulin toxin acts by decreasing sweat, oil, and sebum production.[18,19] Improvement of the appearance of open pores, acne, rosacea, and fine lines are perceived without paralysis of deep muscles.

With the uniform and superficial delivery made possible by the microneedling device, the authors use botulin toxin to promote the microbotox effect.

Indeed, a faster change of the appearance of the skin was perceived when compared with nanofat delivery only. Thus, the use of botulin toxin provided a short-term result while nanofat regenerative capacities were still not perceivable.

Skin booster

Similarly, the authors use a skin booster HA, Belotero Hydro (Merz Aesthetics, Germany), in the mixture with nanofat, botulin toxin, and vitamin C to obtain a short-term enhancement of skin quality before the effect of the nanofat kicks in. The ability of HA to moisturize the skin by attracting water to the tissues is well-known.[20,21] Also, antioxidant effects of HA have been associated with local stimulation of collagen production and regenerative properties.[22,23]

Clinically, a better overall quality of the skin is perceived shortly after the microneedling procedure. After only 5 to 7 days, petechiae produced by the microneedling are gone and patients experience a difference in their skin quality. The authors think that botulin toxin and HA together, rather than just 1 of them, play a role in these short-term changes in skin condition.

Vitamin C

Vitamin C is also added to the mixture together with nanofat, botulin toxin, and HA filler. In vitro and in vivo studies have shown that, when added into the media, vitamin C enhances the viability, survival, and regenerative potential of ADSCs in a dose-dependent manner.[24–27] Also, it is an antioxidant agent that acts as photoprotection from ultraviolet A and B, treatment of hyperpigmentation, and is an important cofactor in collagen synthesis.[28,29] By delivering all these elements to the skin, the authors aim to address a wide range of the structural changes of the aging skin process.

Nanofat cream

Although channels remain open for 30 minutes after needling,[30] a higher permeability of the skin is reported for up to 40 hours after the procedure (depending on the extent and depth of needling).[31] Therefore, in order to maximize potential benefit from nanofat and the other cofactors, and to moisturize the skin during initial healing, the authors developed nanofat cream, a mixture of 50% of emulsifying cream and 50% of nanofat, which is processed at the end of surgery. Patients are instructed to keep it in the refrigerator and use it 5 to 6 times a day during the healing process (normally 5–7 days).

The emulsifying cream components are

- Emulsifying cetostearyl alcohol type B, 3.6 g
- Macrogol cetostearyl ether, 0.9 g
- White petroleum jelly, 7.5 g
- Liquid paraffin, 3 g
- Purified water ad 50 g.

Nanofat Grafting

For small areas, injection of nanofat is easily performed through fine 27-gauge needles. The aim is to inject it intradermally until a blanching is reached. For dark circles in lower eyelids, the aim is to stay above the orbicularis oculi. Typically, blanching will disappear within the hour after the treatment. In mucosal areas, the submucosal plane is the goal. Injection is performed on withdrawal of the needle in a fan-shaped pattern. The needle can be bent 60° to facilitate manipulation. Typically, 1 mL of nanofat can cover a 1-cm by 1-cm area. A lower eyelid needs an average of 2.5 mL of nanofat.

When nanofat needling is planned, quick tapping motions deliver the 8-mL volume of the vial through thousands of microdroplets. The average time to deliver the full volume of the vial is 20 minutes. The authors estimate that the rate of tapping motions performed during needling is 3 per second. Because each tap creates 20 microchannels, 72,000 microchannels are created during the 20-minute treatment. When the full face, neck, and décolleté are addressed, 1 bottle is used for the face only and another is used for the neck and décolleté. At the end of the nanofat needling, a diffuse punctate bleeding shows that the papillary dermis was reached. The nanofat is then left on the skin for another 10 minutes before cleansing the treated areas with saline. After cleansing, nanofat cream is applied.

POSTOPERATIVE CARE

Both nanofat injection with a fine needle and the nanofat needling cause little downtime. In cases of fine-needle injections, minimal yellowish staining should be expected for the first 7 to 10 days and, in cases of needling, erythema, ecchymosis, and petechiae can persist for 5 to 7 days. During this period, patients are advised to use the nanofat cream 5 to 6 times a day. Cream should be kept in the refrigerator in the meantime. With makeup, patients can easily resume their activities 2 days after the procedure.

EXPECTED OUTCOME AND MANAGEMENT OF COMPLICATIONS

With the use of HA filler, botulin toxin, and microbotox, a short-term improvement of skin quality can be perceived after only 2 weeks. The regenerative capacity of the nanofat by itself is expected

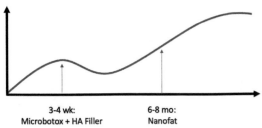

Fig. 2. Clinical perception of increase in skin quality when combining treatments.

3-4 wk:
Microbotox + HA Filler

6-8 mo:
Nanofat

to take 6 to 8 months to be clinically perceivable (**Fig. 2**). Long-term benefit has been observed from the delivery of living SVF cells into the skin.

REVISION OR SUBSEQUENT PROCEDURES

For the treatment of dark circles under the eyes, subsequent procedures may be necessary. In the authors' early series, we had a few cases with persistent yellowish discoloration of the sites of injection for which a corrective procedure with laser resurfacing was needed. This was probably due to inadequate emulsification and incomplete destruction of adipocytes. After the introduction of the 2-step emulsification process followed by filtering, there were no new cases. This mechanical protocol is essential to destroy all the adipocytes and to prevent this complication.

CASE DEMONSTRATIONS
Case 1

See **Fig. 3**.

Case 2

See **Fig. 4.**

Case 3

See **Fig. 5.**

Case 4

See **Fig. 6.**

Case 5

See **Fig. 7.**

DISCUSSION

As the awareness of the structural changes of the skin aging process came to light, the new frontier in rejuvenation became the search and development of new tools to address and reverse these changes. Resurfacing procedures, such as ablative lasers and peelings, have been implemented in the practice of many surgeons; however, the risk of persistent erythema, postinflammatory hyperchromia, permanent hypopigmentation, or (even worse) scars may limit their use, especially in Fitzpatrick skin types III to V. Another limiting factor is their considerably long downtime and recovery period.

The wide availability and ease of processing the fat and the striking clinical results after 6 to 8 months of the treatment have stimulated a shift from ablative therapies to a more regenerative approach. Limited side effects and absence of

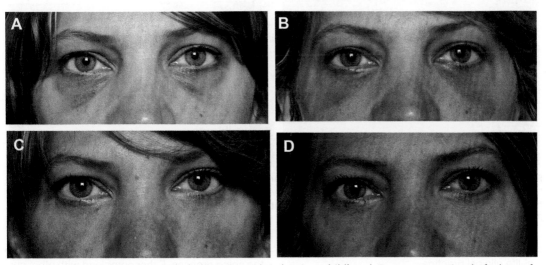

Fig. 3. (*A*) A 33-year-old patient with dark pigmented circles since childhood. Treatment consisted of a lower fat redraping blepharoplasty though a subciliary approach and 1.6 mL of nanofat injection into each pigmented region. (*B*) At 4 months postoperatively, moderate erythema is still present. (*C*) At 7 months postoperatively, redness has disappeared. (*D*) At 5 years postoperatively, the appearance remains stable. (*From* Tonnard P. Centrofacial Rejuvenation. Pg 122–23. Thieme: New York. 2017.)

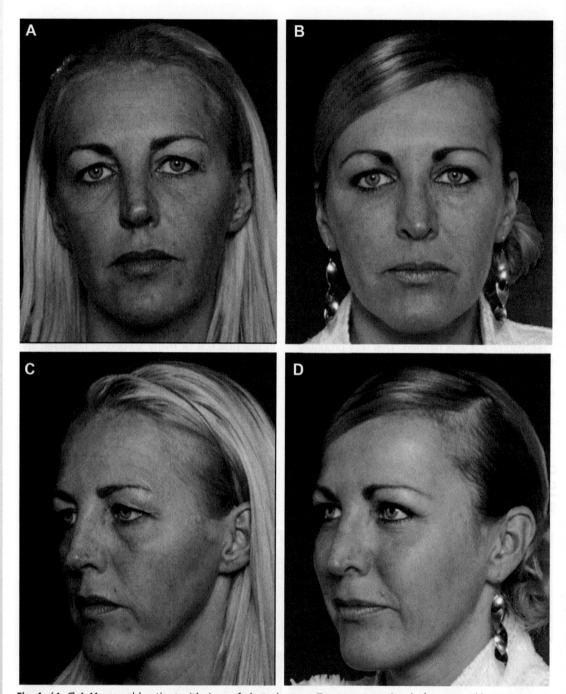

Fig. 4. (*A, C*) A 41-year-old patient with signs of photodamage. Treatment consisted of upper and lower augmentation blepharoplasty and full-face nanofat needling (with botulin toxin). (*B, D*) At 12 months postoperatively, noticeable improvement of quality of skin and pigmentation is seen. (*From* Tonnard P. Centrofacial Rejuvenation. Pg 122–23. Thieme: New York. 2017.)

contraindications bring antiaging medicine into real-life clinical practice.

Clinically, the combination of the power of nanofat with the other described treatment modalities has shown an obvious short-term enhancement of the quality of skin. This encourages clinicians in taking a more proactive posture with regard to the aging process. Either combined with other surgical rejuvenation procedures or alone, nanofat is a tool for plastic surgeons not only looking to reverse structural changes of the aging skin but also looking to prevent them.

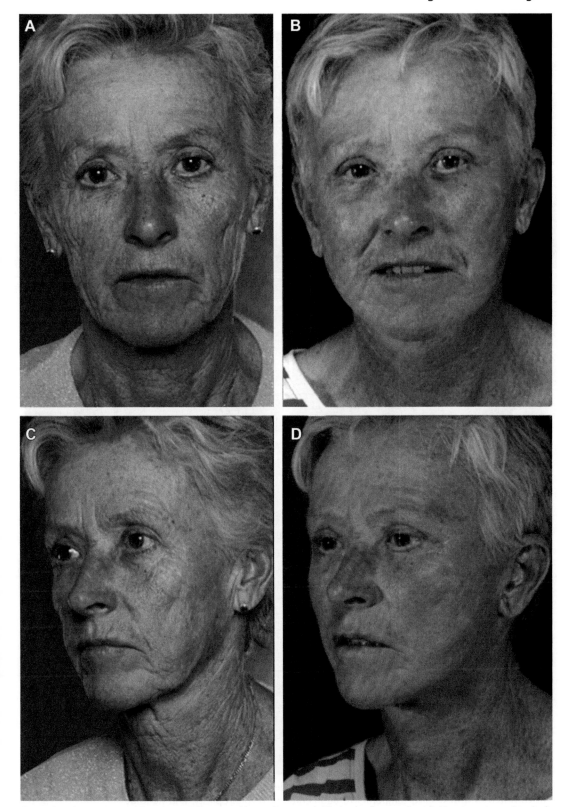

Fig. 5. (*A, C*) A 65-year-old patient with craquelé sun-damaged skin in the face and neck. Treatment consisted of a MACS-lift, temporal-lift, centrofacial lipofilling, and nanofat needling to face and neck. (*B, D*) At 6 months post-operatively, noticeable improvement of quality of skin and pigmentation is seen. MACS, Minimal Access Cranial Suspension.

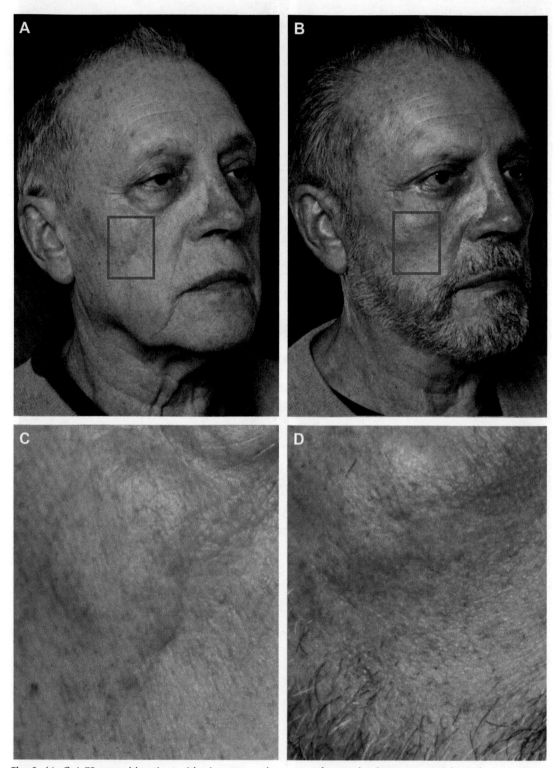

Fig. 6. (*A, C*) A 72-year-old patient with pigmentary changes on face and a deep scar on right malar area. Treatment consisted of a MACS-lift, temporal-lift, augmentation blepharoplasty, and nanofat injections to scar on right malar area. (*B, D*) At 12 months postoperatively, improvement of quality of skin and pigmentation, as well as softening of the scar is noticeable.

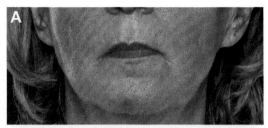
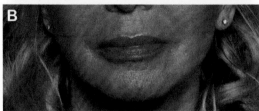

Fig. 7. (*A*) Perioral rejuvenation. A 65-year-old patient with trophic skin changes over the perioral region. Treatment consisted of a MACS-lift and perioral microfat, SNIF, and nanofat injections. (*B*) At 8 years follow-up, noticeable improvement of quality of skin and is seen. SNIF; Sharp Needle Intradermal Fat grafting.

SUMMARY

The cumulative regenerative properties of nanofat encourages clinicians to offer patients an annual or biannual boost of regenerative cells to halt or even reverse the structural changes of the aging skin. Nevertheless, further studies and longer follow-ups are needed. The potential new applications of nanofat are vast.

SUPPLEMENTARY DATA

Supplementary data related to this article can be found online at https://doi.org/10.1016/j.cps.2019.08.006.

REFERENCES

1. Zuk PA, Zhu M, Mizuno H, et al. Multilineage cells from human adipose tissue: implications for cell-based therapies. Tissue Eng 2001;7(2):211–28.
2. Tonnard P, Verpaele A, Peeters G, et al. Nanofat grafting: basic research and clinical applications. Plast Reconstr Surg 2013;132(4):1017–26.
3. Uyulmaz S, Sanchez Macedo N, Rezaeian F, et al. Nanofat grafting for scar treatment and skin quality improvement. Aesthet Surg J 2018;38(4):421–8.
4. Gaur M, Dobke M, Lunyak VV. Mesenchymal stem cells from adipose tissue in clinical applications for dermatological indications and skin aging. Int J Mol Sci 2017;18(1) [pii:E208].
5. Alexander RW. Understanding Adipose-Derived Stromal Vascular Fraction (SVF) Cell Biology in Reconstructive and Regenerative Applications on the Basis of Mononucleated Cell components. Journal of Prolotherapy 2013;10:15–29.
6. Banyard DA, Sarantopoulos CN, Borovikova AA, et al. Phenotypic analysis of stromal vascular fraction after mechanical shear reveals stress-induced progenitor populations. Plast Reconstr Surg 2016;138(2):237e–47e.
7. Charles-de-Sa L, Gontijo-de-Amorim NF, Maeda Takiya C, et al. Antiaging treatment of the facial skin by fat graft and adipose-derived stem cells. Plast Reconstr Surg 2015;135(4):999–1009.
8. Kim DW, Jeon BJ, Hwang NH, et al. Adipose-derived stem cells inhibit epidermal melanocytes through an interleukin-6-mediated mechanism. Plast Reconstr Surg 2014;134(3):470–80.
9. Bertheuil N, Chaput B, Menard C, et al. Adipose mesenchymal stromal cells: definition, immunomodulatory properties, mechanical isolation and interest for plastic surgery. Ann Chir Plast Esthet 2019;64(1):1–10.
10. Jan SN, Bashir MM, Khan FA, et al. Unfiltered nanofat injections rejuvenate postburn scars of face. Ann Plast Surg 2019;82(1):28–33.
11. Xu P, Yu Q, Huang H, et al. Nanofat increases dermis thickness and neovascularization in photoaged nude mouse skin. Aesthetic Plast Surg 2018;42(2):343–51.
12. Cohen SR, Hewett S, Ross L, et al. Regenerative cells for facial surgery: biofilling and biocontouring. Aesthet Surg J 2017;37(suppl_3):S16–32.
13. Caggiati A, Germani A, Di Carlo A, et al. Naturally adipose stromal cell-enriched fat graft: comparative polychromatic flow cytometry study of fat harvested by barbed or blunt multihole cannula. Aesthet Surg J 2017;37(5):591–602.
14. Alharbi Z, Oplander C, Almakadi S, et al. Conventional vs. micro-fat harvesting: how fat harvesting technique affects tissue-engineering approaches using adipose tissue-derived stem/stromal cells. J Plast Reconstr Aesthet Surg 2013;66(9):1271–8.
15. Verpaele A, Tonnard P, Jeganathan C, et al. Nanofat needling: a novel method for uniform delivery of adipose derived stromal vascular fraction into the skin. Plast Reconstr Surg 2019;143(4):1062–5.
16. Ramaut L, Hoeksema H, Pirayesh A, et al. Microneedling: where do we stand now? A systematic review of the literature. J Plast Reconstr Aesthet Surg 2018;71(1):1–14.
17. Tonnard P, Verpaele A, Bensimone R. Centrofacial rejuvenation, vol. III. New York: Thieme; 2017.
18. Wu WT. Microbotox of the lower face and neck: evolution of a personal technique and its clinical effects. Plast Reconstr Surg 2015;136(5 Suppl):92s–100s.
19. Rose AE, Goldberg DJ. Safety and efficacy of intradermal injection of botulinum toxin for the treatment of oily skin. Dermatol Surg 2013;39(3 Pt 1):443–8.

20. Bukhari SNA, Roswandi NL, Waqas M, et al. Hyaluronic acid, a promising skin rejuvenating biomedicine: a review of recent updates and pre-clinical and clinical investigations on cosmetic and nutricosmetic effects. Int J Biol Macromol 2018;120(Pt B):1682–95.

21. Seok J, Hong JY, Choi SY, et al. A potential relationship between skin hydration and stamp-type microneedle intradermal hyaluronic acid injection in middle-aged male face. J Cosmet Dermatol 2016;15(4):578–82.

22. Wang F, Garza LA, Kang S, et al. In vivo stimulation of de novo collagen production caused by cross-linked hyaluronic acid dermal filler injections in photodamaged human skin. Arch Dermatol 2007;143(2):155–63.

23. Turlier V, Delalleau A, Casas C, et al. Association between collagen production and mechanical stretching in dermal extracellular matrix: in vivo effect of cross-linked hyaluronic acid filler. A randomised, placebo-controlled study. J Dermatol Sci 2013;69(3):187–94.

24. Li Y, Zhang W, Chang L, et al. Vitamin C alleviates aging defects in a stem cell model for Werner syndrome. Protein Cell 2016;7(7):478–88.

25. Zhang P, Li J, Qi Y, et al. Vitamin C promotes the proliferation of human adipose-derived stem cells via p53-p21 pathway. Organogenesis 2016;12(3):143–51.

26. Kang KK, Lee EJ, Kim YD, et al. Vitamin C improves therapeutic effects of adipose-derived stem cell transplantation in mouse tendonitis model. In Vivo 2017;31(3):343–8.

27. Kim JH, Kim WK, Sung YK, et al. The molecular mechanism underlying the proliferating and preconditioning effect of vitamin C on adipose-derived stem cells. Stem Cells Dev 2014;23(12):1364–76.

28. Chawla S. Split face comparative study of microneedling with PRP versus microneedling with vitamin C in treating atrophic post acne scars. J Cutan Aesthet Surg 2014;7(4):209–12.

29. Farris PK. Topical vitamin C: a useful agent for treating photoaging and other dermatologic conditions. Dermatol Surg 2005;31(7 Pt 2):814–7 [discussion: 818].

30. Sasaki GH. Micro-needling depth penetration, presence of pigment particles, and fluorescein-stained platelets: clinical usage for aesthetic concerns. Aesthet Surg J 2017;37(1):71–83.

31. Gupta J, Gill HS, Andrews SN, et al. Kinetics of skin resealing after insertion of microneedles in human subjects. J Control Release 2011;154(2):148–55.

Fat Grafting for Facial Rejuvenation with Cryopreserved Fat Grafts

Masanori Ohashi, MD, PhD

KEYWORDS

- Fat grafting • Cryopreservation • Facial rejuvenation • Serial injection • Tissue augmentation

KEY POINTS

- Fat grafting to the face is useful for facial rejuvenation because that procedure can return the patients' facial volume back to the state when they were young and is effective not only for volume augmentation but also for skin rejuvenation.
- Obstacles to fat grafting include the unpredictable maintenance rate for volume augmentation and the unpredictable number of treatments needed to obtain a satisfactory skin rejuvenation effect. Therefore, many patients need repeat sessions.
- Serial fat grafting with fresh fat imposes a burden on the patient not only because of the pain but also because of the downtime of harvest part. If the fat can be preserved and used many times at 1 harvesting, those burdens can be reduced.
- The quality of the fat after cryopreserving and thawing in the proper way is enough for clinical use. The cryopreserved fat could be a new option for serial fat grafting for facial rejuvenation.

INTRODUCTION

One of the biggest reasons for an aging face is the loss of facial volume in both the bony and soft tissues. Since Coleman published the report on "structural fat grafting," fat grafting has become popular, and many investigators confirmed the utility of fat grafting for facial rejuvenation.[1–4] Fat grafting is thought to be an ideal method for facial rejuvenation because it is effective not only for volume augmentation but also for improving skin quality.[5,6]

However, the main problem associated with fat grafting for volume augmentation is the unpredictable volume retention rate. Consequently, it may not be enough with only 1 operation. Therefore, serial injections are often needed to reach the ideal volume and obtain an effective outcome.[7,8] In addition, fat grafting requires fat harvesting, which is painful for patients and time-consuming for surgeons. Therefore, it is ideal if the surgeon can use the fat many times in 1 harvesting.

Although many researchers have concluded that cryopreservation of fat is useful under good conditions,[9,10] almost all such studies were experimental. Very few articles have described the clinical use of fat grafting with cryopreserved fat; moreover, those articles contained a very small number of patients.[11,12]

In this article, the author demonstrates the outcome and ascertains the safety and efficacy of cryopreserved fat for facial rejuvenation based on 173 patients.

SPECIAL CONSIDERATIONS FOR CRYOPRESERVATION OF THE FAT

The author informs the patient of the fact that the rate of maintaining fat grafting is still uncertain, so patients may need serial injections for a

Disclosure Statement: The author has nothing to disclose.
Aesthetic and Plastic Department, THE CLINIC Tokyo, 3-16-23 Nishiazabu Minato-ku, Tokyo 106-0031, Japan
E-mail address: ohashi@theclinic.jp

Clin Plastic Surg 47 (2020) 63–71
https://doi.org/10.1016/j.cps.2019.08.007

satisfied result. Then, the author suggests an alternative option, that the remaining fat can be cryopreserved and stored and used again without reharvesting. If the patient wishes for a serial fat injection with cryopreserved fat, the author explains that we can harvest more fat than can be used at 1 time and cryopreserve the remaining fat.

Only patients who provided written informed consent regarding postoperative infection, inflammation, oil cysts, allergy, fat necrosis, and other potential complications were included in the study. Patients aged less than 19 years and those with diabetes and severe malignant disease were excluded. Consent is obtained that the fat cannot be cryopreserved and stored for anyone who is affected with human immunodeficiency virus, hepatitis C virus, hepatitis B virus, and other severe blood infections.

In Japan, the Act on the Safety of Regenerative Medicine (Regenerative Medicine Safety Act) came into effect as of November 25, 2014 under an institutional framework for promoting the implementation of regenerative medicine. This act, which covers clinical research and private practice, stipulates 3 risk-dependent standards and the procedures for notification of plans for regenerative medicine as well as the standards of cell culture and processing facilities and the licensing procedures to ensure the safety of regenerative medicine.

In accordance with this act, CellSource Co, Ltd (Tokyo, Japan; Certification Number: FA3160006) has been certified as a cell processing center (CPC) by the Ministry of Health, Labor, and Welfare of Japan. In addition, fat grafting with the fat which is centrifuged and/or cryopreserved in a certified facility is approved in Japan (**Fig. 1**).

SURGICAL PROCEDURE
Anesthesia

Most patients were sedated by intravenous anesthesia and provided local anesthesia by a tumescent technique, but without intubation. No patient was under general anesthesia with intubation during surgery.

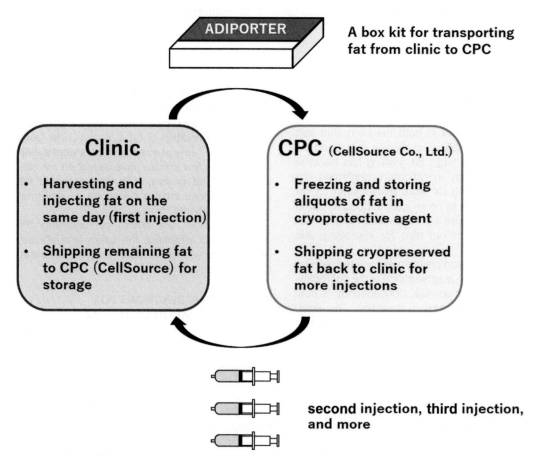

Fig. 1. The flow of harvesting in a clinic and injection of cryopreserved fat.

Harvesting

For fat grafting, the author collected fat by using a tumescent technique (1 mL epinephrine, 20 mL 8.4% sodium hydrogen carbonate, and 50 mL 1.0% lidocaine per 1000 mL of saline solution). The liposuction pressure was set between approximately 70 kPa and 50 kPa.

Donor Sites

The first choices of donor sites were areas of the thighs and (lower) abdominal flank waist (so-called localized fat deposit), according to Geissler and colleagues[13]; the author also deems those parts as being easy to harvest and to cause less bleeding.

Injection on the Same Day of Harvesting (First Injection)

The harvested fat was usually used on the same day as tissue augmentation surgery for facial rejuvenation and/or revitalization/fertilization. In patients who underwent volume augmentation, the author applied the Coleman technique[1,2] (centrifuge 1200g for 3 minutes), and for skin texture rejuvenation (revitalization/fertilization), the author applied the nanofat[3] technique (emulsified fat) or squeezed fat.[14]

The detailed injection technique is in accordance with other investigators; however, the main injection parts for volume augmentation for rejuvenation were (1) forehead and temporal; (2) malar; (3) cheek; (4) nasolabial fold; (5) labiomandibular fold; (6) lips; (7) upper eyelid; (8) lower eyelid; (9) chin. And for skin texture, (1) around the lips; (2) lower eyelid; (3) wrinkles, such as between the eyebrows, forehead, and crow's foot, at the author's institution.

Sending the Collected Fat

The residual fat of the first injection was transferred into the transport bag (FB-bag; CellSource Co, Ltd), which contains an adipose tissue transport medium, is packed in a box called the Adiporter (CellSource Co, Ltd), and is then sent to the CPC at CellSource Co, Ltd in a refrigerated state (<10°C; **Fig. 2**).

Fat Cryopreservation and Storage

The fat-storage processing was performed in the CPC of CellSource Co, Ltd. In brief, the total fat tissue was washed with enough volume of Ringer's lactate solution and centrifuged at 470 g for 3 minutes. The washed fat was rocked with same volume of cryoprotective solution for at least 15 minutes. After removal of the excess cryoprotectant, 4 to 5 mL of the cryoprotectant incorporated fat was transferred to cryovials. The cryovials were cooled at 1°C per minute in a controlled rate freezer to −80°C. Then, for long-term storage, cryopreserved fat was transferred to the liquid nitrogen tank and stored at −196°C. Consequently, the author can make many samples in 1 trip (**Fig. 3**).

Regarding the process of cryopreserving and storage, in the initial stage, CellSource Co, Ltd followed procedures of the American CryoStem Corp. However, CellSource Co, Ltd has changed the protocol of processing and uses their own processing method. Concerning cryoprotective solution, they used ACSelerate-CP (American CryoStem) before, but now they use their own cryoprotective solution because they would like to improve the cell survival rate.

Recall of the Fat

After recalling the required amount of fat through the Internet Web-ordering service of CellSource,

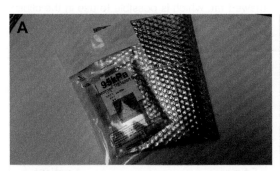
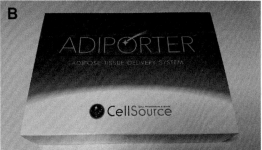

Fig. 2. Transport materials. (*A*) FB-bag (CellSource Co, Ltd), which contains an adipose tissue transport medium. (*B*) Adiporter (CellSource Co, Ltd), which is the box kit for transportation. The fat was sent in the Adiporter to the CPC at CellSource Co, Ltd in a refrigerated state (<10°C). (*From* [*A*, *B*] Ohashi M, Chiba A, Nakai H, et al. Serial injections of cryopreserved fat at -196°C for tissue rejuvenation, scar treatment, and volume augmentation. Plast Reconstr Surg Glob Open. 2018;18(5):e1742; with permission.)

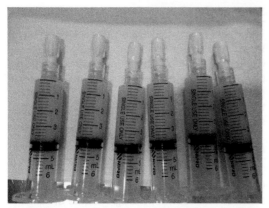

Fig. 3. The collected fat is divided into 4-mL syringes at CellSource Co, Ltd as shown. Consequently, they can make many samples in 1 trip. This picture was taken after cryopreservation and thawing and returned our clinic. It looks fresh, and there is almost no oil in those syringes. (*From* Ohashi M, Chiba A, Nakai H, et al. Serial injections of cryopreserved fat at -196°C for tissue rejuvenation, scar treatment, and volume augmentation. Plast Reconstr Surg Glob Open. 2018;18(5):e1742; with permission.)

the cryopreserved fat was thawed rapidly at 37°C for 6 to 10 minutes in the CPC of CellSource. After thawing, the cryoprotective agents of the fat were washed out with flush centrifuge at 470 g. The recovered fat was filled in small syringes (usually a 5 mL syringe and containing about 4 mL fat) and sent to the author's institution in a refrigerated state (<10°C).

Injection of Cryopreserved Fat

When the author received the fat, he injected it as soon as possible, ideally within 48 hours of being sent to the institution. As for the first injection, the author basically applied the Coleman technique, and for skin texture rejuvenation (revitalization/fertilization), he applied the nanofat (emulsified) technique. The same body parts were not necessarily injected; for example, if the first injection is for the forehead, then, for the second time, the author can inject to the chin.

Repeat Injections

The author can recall the cryopreserved fat again through the Internet service of CellSource Co, Ltd, if residual fat was present. This system allows for serial fat injections for treatment.

ADDITIONAL STUDIES FOR CRYOPRESERVED FAT
Stromal Vascular Fraction Count

The author counted the number of stromal vascular fractions (SVF) in the cryopreserved and

thawed fat before injecting into 5 patients. The SVF was isolated by washing and digested by collagenase (Wako Pure Chemical, Osaka, Japan) for 30 minutes at 37°C in a shaking water bath. Cell numbers and viability of SVF were measured with an automated cell counter (LUNA-STEM Automated Fluorescence Cell Counter; Logos Biosystems, South Korea).

Histologic Analysis of Cryopreserved Fat

The returned fat tissues obtained from the same donor were fixed with 10% formaldehyde for histologic analysis with hematoxylin and eosin (H&E) staining.

POSTOPERATIVE CARE

Basically, postoperative care of cryopreserved fat is the same as for fresh fat.

Namely, after fat grafting (fresh and cryopreserved), one should avoid tight compression with bandages or massages.

Regarding the next fat grafting to the same area with cryopreserved fat, one should wait at least 3 months, because the remodeling of the injected fat continues for 3 months.[15]

For better results, a waiting period of 6 months is generally recommended to allow for initial swelling and resorption to subside.[16]

EXPECTED OUTCOME AND MANAGEMENT OF COMPLICATIONS

Table 1 shows the number of injections per person. **Table 2** shows the ways in which the cryopreserved fat was used. The injection volume ranged from 0.2 to 24.0 mL for the face.

No complications occurred by fat grafting with cryopreserved fat, such as infection, fat necrosis, or similar conditions, for all patients.

In regards to the returned fat (cryopreserved and thawed fat, which is possible to use in the clinic),

Table 1 Number of injection times using cryopreserved fat for the same patient as facial rejuvenation	
1 time	173 patients
2 times	42 patients
3 times	17 patients
4 times	7 patients
5 times	1 patient

One time means the first injection of fresh fat and cryopreserved fat was used 1 time. In the same manner, for example, 2 times means the first injection of fresh fat and cryopreserved fat was used 2 times.

Table 2 The ways to use their cryopreserved fat (same patient might be injected many places) as facial rejuvenation	
Facial Rejuvenation	Total 173 Patients
For volume augmentation only (use cryopreserved fat as it is)	155 cases
For skin rejuvenation only (use cryopreserved fat as nanofat/squeezed fat)	13 cases
For volume augmentation and skin rejuvenation	72 cases

As for volume augmentation, 3 main parts were the forehead, malar, and nasolabial fold. As for skin rejuvenation, the main parts were in the region of the lips, lower eyelids, and wrinkles, such as crow's feet.

the rate that compares to send-out volume was 34.4% ± 5.5% if sent without centrifuging, and 51.3% ± 9.8% if the fat is already centrifuged (**Table 3**).

The mean number of SVF in the cryopreserved (returned) fat was 14.8×10^5/mL compared with 7.1×10^5/mL of sent fat (n = 5); therefore, returned fat contains about double the amount of SVF.

Regarding histologic analysis of cryopreserved (returned) fat, before and after tissues were found to be very similar (**Fig. 4**).

REVISION OR SUBSEQUENT PROCEDURES

Concerning revision or subsequent procedures for fat grafting with cryopreserved fat, it is same as fat grafting with fresh fat. The author has not experienced any special complication for cryopreserved fat.

Of course, in case one has cryopreserved fat, additional fat grafting is easy for revision. Thus,

Table 3 Volume change of fat after cryopreservation		
	Not Centrifuged (n = 16)	Centrifuged (n = 60)
Sent volume, mL	205 ± 86.3	167 ± 79.5
Returned volume, mL	71 ± 35.5	76 ± 43.9
% volume	34.7 ± 7.9	57.8 ± 9.5

Not centrifuged means only gravity, and centrifuged means 700 to 1200*g* for 3 min.
Returned volume means cryopreserved and thawed fat, which is possible to use in the clinic.

storing the fat as cryopreserved fat is useful for the patient's satisfaction.

CASE DEMONSTRATIONS
Case 1

A 46-year-old woman reported that she was bothered by her thin and aging face (**Fig. 5**). She underwent facial rejuvenation surgery involving fat grafting of the forehead, cheeks, and lips with a thread lift. She was concerned about the downtime involved with liposuction, and she cryopreserved her fat at −196°C. After her first injection, she underwent 2 cryopreserved fat-grafting sessions in about 1 year. She appeared younger and healthy after these treatments.

Case 2

A 47-year-old woman reported that she was bothered by her hollow of forehead and aging face (**Fig. 6**). She underwent facial fat grafting of the forehead, malar, cheeks, upper and lower eyelids, and chin with lower orbital fat removal. After her first injection, she received cryopreserved fat-grafting sessions 2 times in 2 years. A postoperative photograph is 3.5 years after the first injection and 1 year after the last session. However, her forehead is still round, and her face looks younger than 3.5 years ago.

Case 3

A 60-year-old woman reported that she was bothered by her tired-looking face (**Fig. 7**). She underwent facial fat grafting of the forehead, malar, nasolabial fold, labiomandibular fold, and chin, with a thread lift. After her first injection, she received cryopreserved fat-grafting sessions after half a year. The postoperative photograph is 1 year after the first injection and a half year after the second injection; however, her face appears much younger than before the operation.

DISCUSSION

Both plastic surgeons and patients have expressed a strong desire to preserve adipose tissue.

On the other hand, as for cost of on the clinic side (especially for the small clinic), preserving the fat at −196°C might be difficult because of the high costs of making CPC and purchasing expensive equipment, such as program-freezer.

Therefore, the author chose to send the fat to the specialized company, and the company cryopreserves the fat in their CPC. Then, a small clinic can preserve the fat without a high initial

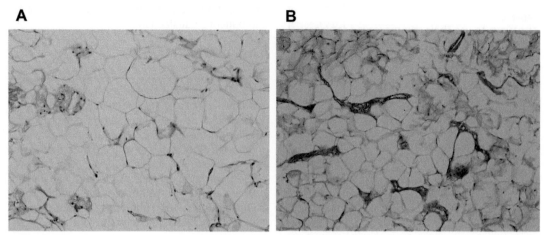

Fig. 4. Histologic analysis of the fat tissue before and after cryopreservation and thawing. The fat tissues obtained from the same donor were fixed with 10% formaldehyde for histologic analysis with H&E staining (×200). (*A*) The tissue processed without freezing. (*B*) The tissue that cryopreserved at −196°C and thawed. Both tissues were found to be very similar. (*From* Ohashi M, Chiba A, Nakai H, et al. Serial injections of cryopreserved fat at -196°C for tissue rejuvenation, scar treatment, and volume augmentation. Plast Reconstr Surg Glob Open. 2018;18(5):e1742; with permission.)

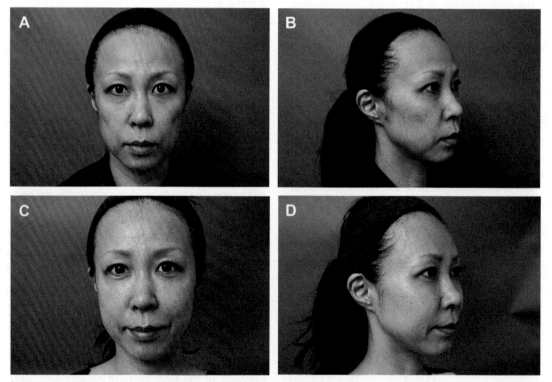

Fig. 5. Case 1: Facial rejuvenation with cryopreserved fat grafting. A 46-year-old woman received 1 fresh fat grafting (forehead, lower eyelids, cheeks, and lips) with thread lift. After her first injection, she received cryopreserved fat grafting 3 times to her forehead, lower eyelids, cheeks, and lips. (*A*) Preoperation (front view of face). (*B*) Preoperation (diagonal view of face). (*C*) Six months after second cryopreserved fat grafting (front view of face). (*D*) Six months after second cryopreserved fat grafting (diagonal view of face). (*From [A, C]* Ohashi M, Chiba A, Nakai H, et al. Serial injections of cryopreserved fat at -196°C for tissue rejuvenation, scar treatment, and volume augmentation. Plast Reconstr Surg Glob Open. 2018;18(5):e1742; with permission.)

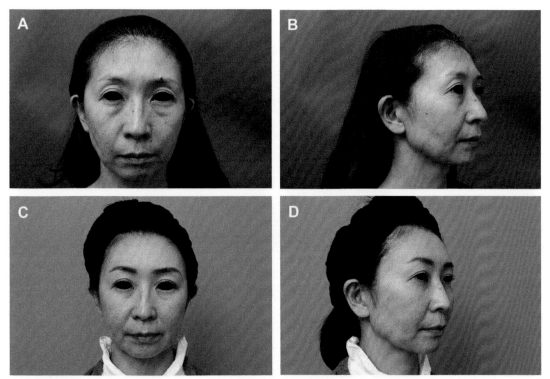

Fig. 6. Case 2: Facial rejuvenation with cryopreserved fat grafting. A 47-year-old woman reported that she was bothered by her hollow forehead and aging face. She underwent facial fat grafting of the forehead, malar, cheeks, upper and lower eyelids, and chin with lower orbital fat removal. After her first injection, she received cryopreserved fat grafting sessions 2 times in 2 years. Postoperative photograph is 3.5 years after first injection and 1 year after last session; however, forehead is still round and her face looks younger than 3.5 years ago. (*A*) Preoperation (front view of face). (*B*) Preoperation (diagonal view of face). (*C*) Postoperation (front view of face). (*D*) Postoperation (diagonal view of face).

investment and maintenance cost. For example, the author's present protocol involved sending the harvested fat to CellSource Co, Ltd, and they cryopreserved the fat in their CPC. This system (see **Fig. 1**) made it easy to perform safer preservation without technical or financial difficulties.

The cases the author has presented have shown that this method, in which the fat is sent to an external company that cryopreserves it with an adequate method and then the fat is recalled, works well for serial injections (cases 1–3) and is a useful way to use residual fat for another parts (eg, first for facial rejuvenation, second for hand rejuvenation). Thus, the author believes that this is a very easy method of serial fat grafting and use of residual fat, even in small clinics.

Concerning the cryopreservation of fat, it has been controversial because of viability and safety concerns. Many investigators recently suggested that if an adequate cryopreservation technique is used, high fat viability can be achieved.[9,11,17–19]

The great concerns during cryopreservation are freezing temperature, cooling and thawing temperature, and the use of cryoprotective agents.[9,11,18,19]

The author's present protocol involved sending the harvested fat to CellSource Co, Ltd, and they cryopreserved the fat in their CPC. This process made it easy to perform safer preservation without technical or financial difficulties (eg, to make CPC).

Adipose-derived stem cells play a role in the regeneration of grafted fat and contribute to the survival rate of fat grafting.[20] Also, the adipose-derived stem cells have a stronger response to stresses, such as ischemia, transportation (mechanical damage), and cryopreservation, than do mature adipocytes.

As a result, the fat volume, which the author sent, decreased 34% (if sent without centrifuge), and 51% (if already centrifuged) when received. Consequently, the volume of the fat returned to the clinic is smaller than that sent out from the clinic. This is one of the disadvantages of this system.

On the other hand, the mean number of SVF in the cryopreserved (returned) fat was

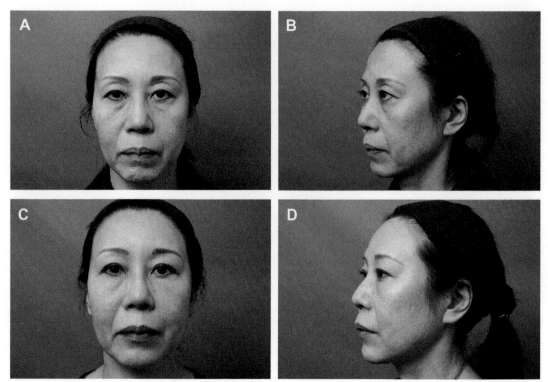

Fig. 7. Case 3: Facial rejuvenation with cryopreserved fat grafting. A 60-year-old woman reported that she was bothered by her tired-looking face. She underwent facial fat grafting of the forehead, malar, nasolabial fold, labiomandibular fold, and chin, with a thread lift. After her first injection, she received cryopreserved fat-grafting sessions after a half year. Postoperative photograph is 1 year after the first injection and a half year after second injection; however, her face appears much younger than before the operation. (*A*) Preoperation (front view of face). (*B*) Preoperation (diagonal view of face). (*C*) Postoperation (front view of face). (*D*) Postoperation (diagonal view of face).

14.8×10^5/mL compared with 7.1×10^5/mL of sent fat (n = 5). Consequently, returned fat contains about double the amount of SVF. Thus, cryopreservation could be considered an option for condensing adipocyte-derived stem cells.

In any case, with the present protocol, the amount of adipocyte and SVF was decreased through the process of transportation, freezing, and thawing. As a result, the protocol and technique of cryopreservation should be improved for cell damage.

SUMMARY

The fact that no complications occurred among all 173 patients indicates the safety of serial injection using cryopreserved fat, at least in the short-term follow-up. The author did not compare the retention rate and effect of revitalization/fertilization with those of fresh fat. Further research involving longer follow-up is needed to determine whether cryopreserved fat can serve as a new option for better facial rejuvenation.

REFERENCES

1. Coleman SR. Structural fat grafting: more than a permanent filler. Plast Reconstr Surg 2006;118(Suppl): 108S–20S.
2. Coleman SR, Grover R. The anatomy of the aging face: volume loss and changes in 3-dimensional topography. Aesthet Surg J 2006;26(suppl):S4–9.
3. Tonnard P, Verpaele A, Peeters G, et al. Nanofat grafting: basic research and clinical applications. Plast Reconstr Surg 2013;132:1017.
4. Marten MJ, Elyassnia D. Fat grafting in facial rejuvenation. Clin Plast Surg 2015;42:219–52.
5. Charles-de-Sa L, Gontijo-de-Amorim NF, Takiya CM, et al. Antiaging treatment of the facial skin by fat graft and adipose- derived stem cells. Plast Reconstr Surg 2015;135:999.
6. Mojallal A, Lequeux C, Shipkov C, et al. Improvement of skin quality after fat grafting: clinical observation and an animal study. Plast Reconstr Surg 2009;124:765–74.
7. Losken A, Pinell XA, Sikoro K, et al. Autologous fat grafting in secondary breast reconstruction. Ann Plast Surg 2011;66:518–22.

8. Kim HY, Jung BK, Lew DH, et al. Autologous fat graft in the reconstructed breast: fat absorption rate and safety based on sonographic identification. Arch Plast Surg 2014;41:740–7.

9. Pu LLQ, Coleman SR, Cui X, et al. Cryopreservation of autologous fat grafts harvested with the Coleman technique. Ann Plast Surg 2010;64:337.

10. Gir P, Brown SA, Oni G, et al. Fat grafting: evidence-based review on autologous fat harvesting, processing, reinjection, and storage. Plast Reconstr Surg 2012;130:249–58.

11. Pu LLQ, Cui X, Fink BF, et al. Adipose aspirates as a source for human processed lipoaspirate cells after optimal cryopreservation. Plast Reconstr Surg 2006; 117:1845–50.

12. Ibrahiem SMS, Farouk A, Salem IM. Facial rejuvenation: serial fat graft transfer. Alexandria J Med 2016; 52:371–6.

13. Geissler PJ, Davis K, Roostaeian J, et al. Improving fat transfer viability: the role of aging, body mass index, and harvest site. Plast Reconstr Surg 2014; 134(2):227–32.

14. Mashiko T, Wu SH, Yoshimura K, et al. Mechanical micronization of lipoaspirates: squeeze and emulsification techniques. Plast Reconstr Surg 2017;139:79–90.

15. Kato H, Mineda K, Eto H, et al. Degeneration, regeneration, and cicatrization after fat grafting: dynamic total tissue remodeling during the first 3 months. Plast Reconstr Surg 2014;133:303e.

16. Meier JD, Glasgold RA, Glasgold MJ. Autologous fat grafting; long-term evidence of its efficacy in midfacial rejuvenation. Arch Facial Plast Surg 2009;11(1): 24–8.

17. MacRae JW, Tholapdady SS, Ogale RC, et al. Ex vivo fat graft preservation: effects and implications of cryopreservation. Ann Plast Surg 2004; 52(3):281–2 [discussion: 283].

18. Pu LL. Cryopreservation of adipose tissue. Organogenesis 2009;5(3):138–42.

19. Shu Z, Gao D, Pu LL. Update on cryopreservation of adipose tissue and adipose-derived stem cells. Clin Plast Surg 2015;42(2):209–18.

20. Yoshimura K, Sato K, Aoi N, et al. Cell-assisted lipotransfer (CAL) for cosmetic breast augmentation–supportive use of adipose-derived stem/stromal cells. Aesthetic Plast Surg 2008;32: 48–55.

Fat Grafting for Facial Rejuvenation Using Stromal Vascular Fraction Gel Injection

Shenglu Jiang, MD, Yuping Quan, MD, Jing Wang, MD,
Junrong Cai, MD, PhD*, Feng Lu, MD, PhD*

KEYWORDS

- Fat grafting • Stromal vascular fraction gel • Tear trough deformity • Lower eye bag
- Transconjunctival lower eyelid blepharoplasty

KEY POINTS

- The preferred donor sites for facial fat grafting are the abdomen or thigh.
- Stromal vascular fraction gel (SVF-gel) is prepared by a series of mechanical processes, including centrifugation and intersyringe shifting.
- SVF-gel is particularly rich in SVF cells and native adipose extracellular matrix (ECM).
- SVF-gel injection shows greater therapeutic effect in correcting the palpebromalar groove, tear trough deformity, and periorbital hollow.

 Video content accompanies this article at http://www.plasticsurgery.theclinics.com.

INTRODUCTION

Aesthetic changes of the lower eyelid and midface represent some of the earliest clinically detectable areas of aging on the face. During the aging process, the supporting ligaments and tissues of the face and eyes experience irreversible changes, which combine to create a vertically elongated lower eyelid, a lax lower eyelid and protrusion of orbital fat, and ptotic malar/cheek complex.[1] To eliminate the "tired appearance," the surgeon attempts to reverse aging and gravitational changes in the lid/cheek complex with a goal to shorten that distance and suspend tissues.

For several years, the traditional surgical approach to lower eyelid blepharoplasty was to remove the pseudoherniated orbital fat via a transconjunctival or transcutaneous incision.[2] The transconjunctival lower eyelid blepharoplasty offers an advantageous access to the lower eyelid and midcheek with no trauma to the anterior lamella of the lower eyelid and its quick recovery. However, infraorbital sunken and skeletal appearance of the eye was easily created when excessive orbital fat was excised.[3] Additionally, conventional excision of excess intraorbital fat cannot sufficiently correct contour irregularities and attenuate tear trough deformity.[4]

S. Jiang and Y. Quan contributed equally.

Disclosure: The authors have nothing to disclose.

Funding: This work was supported by National Nature Science Foundation of China (81671931, 81701920), President Foundation of Nanfang Hospital (2016C032), and Administrator Foundation of Nanfang Hospital (2016b001).

Department of Plastic and Cosmetic Surgery, Nanfang Hospital, Southern Medical University, 1838 Guangzhou North Road, Guangzhou, Guangdong 510515, P. R. China

* Corresponding authors.

E-mail addresses: drjunrongcai@outlook.com (J.C.); doctorlufeng@hotmail.com (F.L.)

Clin Plastic Surg 47 (2020) 73–79
https://doi.org/10.1016/j.cps.2019.09.001

To avoid infraorbital hollow, fat repositioning techniques or filling techniques using autologous or nonautologous materials are increasingly applied.[5,6] The advantage of autologous fat grafting to the infraorbital area is achieving midcheek augmentation and improving the palpebromalar groove and addressing the tear trough deformity without disrupting the middle lamellae. However, traditional fat grafting is not an optimal alternative for periorbital injection because it uses particles of fairly large size, which may easily result in uneven skin surface or excess fullness.

In this article, we reported a novel adipose tissue–derived product called stromal vascular fraction gel (SVF-gel) for the purpose of infraorbital injection to correct infraorbital hollow and tear trough. SVF-gel is prepared by a process of centrifugation and intersyringe shifting. It has a smooth texture and is injected though a fine, 27-gauge needle. SVF-gel is particularly rich in SVF cells and native adipose extracellular matrix (ECM).[7] SVF-gel can thus act as a natural filler, because it contains condensed adipose tissue ECM fibers. To validate its promising clinical applications, several case examples are presented to highlight those well-designed steps in fat grafting for facial rejuvenation, especially for the periorbital area.

PREOPERATIVE EVALUATION AND SPECIAL CONSIDERATIONS

Each patient's general health conditions and past medical or surgical history should be reviewed first. The major exclusion criteria includes a history of trauma or other comorbidities, operation, or filler injection in the injection area. Three-dimensional photographs are routinely taken and recorded before the surgical procedure and the individual aging degree especially the gravitational changes in the lid/cheek complex should be carefully evaluated and noted. Because the quality of facial skin and facial anatomy varies from person to person, signs of facial aging, such as soft tissue atrophy, structural ptosis, laxity of skin, and abruptly emerging lines, are analyzed and documented with detail. The potential donor sites for fat grafts harvested should also be carefully examined and marked.

Harvest of fat grafts should be performed under general anesthesia. The tumescent solution used for donor site analgesia and hemostasis should contain the lowest concentration of lidocaine and ropivacaine because their high concentration has been proved to impair the adipocyte function. In general, we use 0.03% of lidocaine and 0.01% of ropivacaine in 500 mL of normal saline. The tumescent solution also contains epinephrine with a concentration of 1:100,000. Epinephrine can precipitate vasoconstriction in the donor sites, which tends to decrease the quantity of blood loss, occurrence of bruising and hematoma, and the possibility of intra-arterial injection of the transplanted fat particles especially when injecting around periorbital or temporal area.

Because SVF-gel is rich in SVF cells and native adipose ECM and the oil drops have been massively wiped off through a process of centrifugation and intersyringe shifting, SVF-gel manifests an obviously higher retention rate than traditionally processed fat grafts after transplantation.[7] The injection volume of SVF-gel mainly depends on the volume depletion of soft tissue based on the preoperative evaluation. Unlike traditional fat grafting, because SVF-gel has a great retention rate of 80%, overcorrection is not necessary in SVF-gel injection.

SURGICAL PROCEDURES
Donor Site Selection

In clinical practice, lower abdomen and inner thigh are the optimal donor sites for fat graft harvest because well-designed suction in these sites could significantly enhance the body contour and they are accessible in the supine position in which facial rejuvenation is performed. Besides, fat reserves in lower abdomen and inner thigh are adequate for the production of SVF-gel. According to published literature, fat grafts harvested from lower abdomen and inner thigh are reported to have higher concentration of adipose-derived stem cells. Thus we routinely choose lower abdomen and inner thigh as the donor sites.

Fat Graft Harvesting

After local anesthesia, incisions should be done in the specified locations where the scar is easily concealed. Usually lower abdomen and inner thigh incisions are symmetric and located on the margin of pubic hair and on the groin, respectively, with the size of 5 to 10 mm. A cylindrical clamp is sutured to the skin to reduce the mechanical trauma during the process of liposuction and to dilate the underlying subcutaneous tissues through the incision to allow insertion of the harvesting cannula. The tumescent solution is then equably infiltrated to the donor sites 10 minutes before fat extraction, which makes harvesting of fat grafts easier to operate with less trauma and makes the patient less painful in the recovery. It should be noted that the tip of the infiltration cannula we specially designed is usually blunt and has multiple oblong openings on the side. Usually a 20-mL Luer-Lok syringe is connected with a harvesting cannula with a 2.5-mm inner diameter for liposuction. This kind of cannula is more efficient for fat extraction. Gentle pulling back on the plunger creates a space vacuum negative pressure in the syringe. With gentle back and forth movement of the assembled syringe, the fat is gradually collected. After harvest, all incision sites are closed with interrupted sutures once excess tumescent fluid is milked out.

Fat Graft Processing

SVF-gel was obtained as previously reported (Video 1).[7] Standard Coleman fat was the product we use to make SVF-gel. The Coleman fat was prepared according to the standard Coleman technique. The lipoaspirate was centrifuged at 1200 × g for 3 minutes to obtain Coleman fat in the middle layer. The bottom layer of the tumescent fluid was discarded, and 20 mL of Coleman fat was transferred to two 20-mL syringes connected by a Luer-Lok connector (internal diameter of 1.4 mm). The Coleman fat was then transferred between two syringes (six to eight times) at a rate of 20 mL/s until the Coleman fat converted into a uniform emulsion, which was then centrifuged at 2000 × g for 3 minutes. The middle layer, which had a volume of approximately 20% of the original Coleman fat, was identified as SVF-gel and collected for further use (**Fig. 1**).

Preparation of Recipient Site

During the process of SVF-gel preparation, transconjunctival eye bag removal was performed. One drop of 0.5% proparacaine hydrochloride ophthalmic solution was instilled in each eye. Because of rich blood supply in the face, the possibility of intravascular injections causing fat embolism to the brain or eye is real and may be avoided when 1% lidocaine with 1:100,000 epinephrine is injected into each medial, central, and lateral intraorbital fat pad adjacent to the conjunctiva for possible vasoconstriction. Adequate compression after injection of the previously mentioned anesthetic solution is needed to minimize swelling so that precise injection of SVF-gel can still be made by the plastic surgeon according to the volume requirement of fat grafts in each area.

An incision was made on the conjunctiva 5 mm below the lower eyelid margin. The eyelid edge of the divided conjunctiva was similarly retracted caudally using a lid retractor. A further incision was made directly on the capsulopalpebral fascia toward the infraorbital fat pads to keep the orbital septum intact, and a retroseptal dissection was performed. After the orbital fat pads were exposed, gentle pressure was placed on the globe to allow the fat to herniate through the incision site. At this point, fat protruding through the incision was carefully excised using the carbon dioxide electrocautery laser. After the planned amount of fat was excised, the divided capsulopalpebral fascia and conjunctiva were returned to their original locations and were left there without suturing.

Injection of Fat Grafts

Patients were then awake and positioned upright for SVF-gel injection. The prepared SVF-gel was transferred to a 1-mL Luer-Lok syringe for injection. Either one or two entry points are made on the lateral end of the palpebromalar groove and extension line of the nasojugal groove. We used a Tulip 0.9-mm blunt-tip injector to inject the SVF-gel into the space between the orbicularis oculimuscle and the infraorbital septum, and the injected materials were diffusely distributed. A cold compress was used to minimize discomfort and swelling and to help contour the skin postoperatively, as tolerated, for the first 48 hours. Regular postoperative care also included the administration of oral antibiotics and nonsteroidal anti-inflammatory drugs for 3 days when necessary.

POSTOPERATIVE CARE

According to our clinical practice, SVF-gel injection in the recipient site usually resulted in mild or no swelling, which disappeared in 1 or 2 weeks. Patients are informed about this normal process after SVF-gel injection.

In the recovery, stretch pants or bellybands are routinely wrapped over the donor sites, whereas the recipient sites should not be applied with much compression when taping. Patients are clearly informed that pressing or touching of the grafted areas should be strictly prohibited.

EXPECTED OUTCOME AND MANAGEMENT OF COMPLICATIONS

From December of 2017 to December of 2018, 32 patients underwent transconjunctival eye bag removal with SVF-gel injection and 42 patients only received SVF-gel injection to correct tear trough deformity or infraorbital hollow. Other concomitant facial procedures performed for the patients during the same operation included upper blepharoplasty, fat grafting, and face lift.

The mean operative time for fat harvest and process was 43 minutes (range, 30–60 minutes). The lower eyelid procedure, if needed, adds 15 to 30 minutes to the procedure. The mean follow-up was 6 months (range, 3–12 months). We have

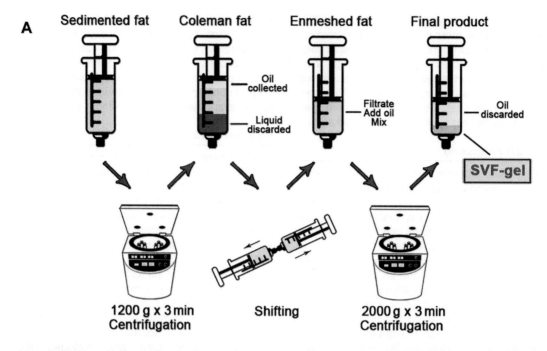

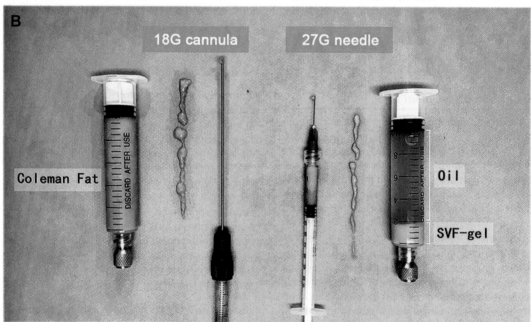

Fig. 1. (*A*) The processing procedure of SVF-gel. (*B*) Centrifuged Coleman fat and SVF-gel after processing. SVF-gel is easily injected through a 27-gauge needle; however, Coleman fat can only pass through an 18-gauge cannula.

used our technique for a range of aging changes and anatomy. The revision rate was 4% (3 of 74); revisions were for reinjection of SVF-gel because of fat absorption.

Rare complications were observed. Two patients had a tiny bulge from a small hematoma around the inferior oblique muscle that resolved in about 2 weeks. No patient experienced chemosis, prolonged swelling, lower eyelid retraction, ectropion, or lumpiness of the grafted fat.

REVISION OR SUBSEQUENT PROCEDURES

In our practice, facial SVF-gel injection is usually performed once for most patients with satisfactory

before

1 y postoperation

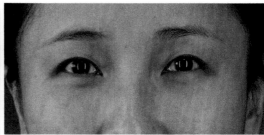

Fig. 2. A 41-year-old woman presented with eye bags and a prominent tear trough deformity. A transconjunctival lower blepharoplasty with SVF-gel injection was performed. She is shown here preoperatively and 1 year postoperatively.

outcome. However, subsequent SVF-gel injection may be needed for some patients if additional injection is necessary to improve clinical outcome.

CASE DEMONSTRATIONS
Case 1

A 41-year-old woman presented with eye bags and a prominent tear trough deformity. A transconjunctival lower blepharoplasty with SVF-gel injection was performed. She is shown here preoperatively and 1 year postoperatively (**Fig. 2**).

Case 2

A 30-year-old woman presented with eye bags and a prominent tear trough deformity. A transconjunctival lower blepharoplasty with SVF-gel injection was performed. She is shown here preoperatively and 1 year postoperatively (**Fig. 3**).

Case 3

A 34-year-old patient presented with tear trough and tired appearance. She received SVF-gel injection. She is shown here preoperatively and 1 year

postoperatively. Note the improvement in the tear trough deformity, giving a fresher and more youthful appearance (**Fig. 4**).

Case 4

A 36-year-old patient presented with tear trough and supraorbital hollow. She received SVF-gel injection to the tear trough and supraorbital area. She is shown here preoperatively and 1 year postoperatively. Note the improvement in the tear trough deformity and supraorbital hollow. Moreover, better skin condition is observed after SVF-gel injection (**Fig. 5**).

DISCUSSION

During the aging process, loss of the supporting ligaments and gravitational shifting of the dermal matrix volume result in the laxity and elongation of the lower eyelid and the protrusion of the orbital fat, which clarify the formation of what is normally called "eye bags."[8] Conventional transconjunctival lower eyelid blepharoplasty techniques are

before

6 mo postoperation

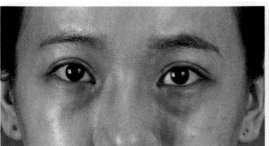
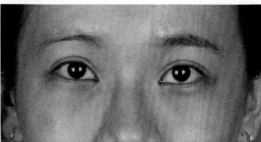

Fig. 3. A 30-year-old woman presented with eye bags and a prominent tear trough deformity. A transconjunctival lower blepharoplasty with SVF-gel injection was performed. She is shown here preoperatively and 1 year postoperatively.

before   6 mo postoperation

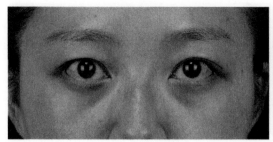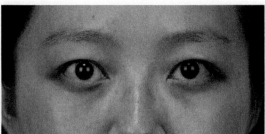

Fig. 4. A 34-year-old woman presented with tear trough and tired appearance. She received SVF-gel injection. She is shown here preoperatively and 1 year postoperatively. Note the improvement in the tear trough deformity, giving a fresher and more youthful appearance.

generally effective for patients with true eye bag fat excess.[9]

However, a skeletonized eye might be created once too much fat is removed, which severely influences the aesthetic effect. To confront this dilemma, autologous fat was frequently used to assist transconjunctival lower eyelid blepharoplasty.[10] Moreover, the autologous fat grafting can also be applied to correct the palpebromalar groove, tear trough deformity, and supraorbital hollow. However, traditional fat grafting has large particle size and cannot ensure precise injection, which may easily lead to uneven surface and noticeable nodule in the periorbital area because the eyelids have thin skin. Unlike traditional fat, SVF-gel is emulsified and is easily injected through a fine, 27-gauge needle, which enables precise injection and avoids appearing as beaded structures.[11] Thus, SVF-gel is suitable for periorbital injection with its smooth texture.

Conventional fat grafts have a high absorption rate. Overcorrection is preferred to increase the retention rate, increasing the volume of fat grafts and contributing to severe postinjection swelling around the orbital area. Our previous studies have demonstrated that SVF-gel grafting has higher retention rate than conventional fat grafting.[7,12] Overcorrection is not necessary for SVF-gel grafting, which enables surgeons to precisely inject the volume that is needed. Moreover, conventional fat grafting frequently involves the use of blunt cannulae of diameter 18-gauge or larger. By contrast, SVF-gel is easily injected through a 25-gauge cannula or 27-gauge needle, causing less tissue damage and attenuating damage-induced inflammation.[13] Thus, SVF-gel grafting does not result in significant swelling after injection. Patients can enjoy a quick recovery period with this technique.

Moreover, improvement on skin was observed in most patients receiving SVF-gel grafting. SVF-gel was previously demonstrated to have higher adipose stem cell (ASC) and other SVF cell density than Coleman fat.[7] In addition, SVF-gel was proved to have excellent efficacy in promoting wound healing and increasing the survival rate of ischemic flaps.[14] ASCs are the key functional cell populations among mesenchymal cell therapy. It was

before   1 y postoperation

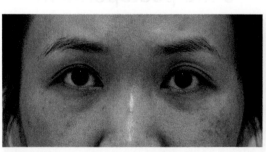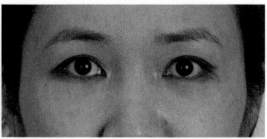

Fig. 5. A 36-year-old woman presented with tear trough and supraorbital hollow. She received SVF-gel injection to the tear trough and supraorbital area. She is shown here preoperatively and 1 year postoperatively. Note the improvement in the tear trough deformity and supraorbital hollow. Moreover, better skin condition is observed after SVF-gel injection.

reported that ASCs can secrete different types of collagen and stimulate the synthesis of collagen by local fibroblasts.[15] Thus, the transplanted SVF-gel has the potential to not only function as a filler, but also to stimulate collagen synthesis by the paracrine effect of ASCs and other SVF cells.[12]

Patient selection should be well considered. In most cases, this technique is preferred for younger patients with aging changes occurring primarily with eye bags, a prominent tear trough deformity, and maxillary retrusion. Patients with severe skin laxity are not a good candidate. The excess skin should be removed with transcutaneous operations in these patients.

SUMMARY

SVF-gel, a mechanically processed adipose tissue–derived product, is precisely injected to periorbital area to assist transconjunctival lower eyelid blepharoplasty and correct the palpebromalar groove, tear trough deformity, and supraorbital hollow.

SUPPLEMENTARY DATA

Supplementary data related to this article can be found online at https://doi.org/10.1016/j.cps.2019.09.001.

REFERENCES

1. Branham GH. Lower eyelid blepharoplasty. Facial Plast Surg Clin North Am 2016;24(2):129–38.
2. Triana RJ, Larrabee WJ. Lower eyelid blepharoplasty: the aging eyelid. Facial Plast Surg 1999; 15(3):203–12.
3. Wang Q, Wang J. Extended transconjunctival lower eyelid blepharoplasty with release of the tear trough ligament and fat redistribution. Plast Reconstr Surg 2018;141(3):441e.
4. Duan R, Wu M, Tremp M, et al. Modified lower blepharoplasty with fat repositioning via transconjunctival approach to correct tear trough deformity. Aesthetic Plast Surg 2019;43(3):680–5.
5. Archibald DJ, Farrior EH. Fat repositioning in lower eyelid blepharoplasty. JAMA Facial Plast Surg 2014;16(5):375–6.
6. Baker SR. Orbital fat preservation in lower-lid blepharoplasty. Arch Facial Plast Surg 1999;1(1):33–7.
7. Yao Y, Dong Z, Liao Y, et al. Adipose extracellular matrix/stromal vascular fraction gel: a novel adipose tissue-derived injectable for stem cell therapy. Plast Reconstr Surg 2017;139(4):867–79.
8. Sand JP, Zhu BZ, Desai SC. Surgical anatomy of the eyelids. Facial Plast Surg Clin North Am 2016;24(2): 89–95.
9. Tessier P. The conjunctival approach to the orbital floor and maxilla in congenital malformation and trauma. J Maxillofac Surg 1973;1(1):3–8.
10. Coleman SR. Lower lid deformity secondary to autogenous fat transfer: a cautionary tale. Aesthetic Plast Surg 2008;32(3):415–7.
11. Yao Y, Cai J, Zhang P, et al. Adipose stromal vascular fraction gel grafting: a new method for tissue volumization and rejuvenation. Dermatol Surg 2018;44(10):1278–86.
12. Zhang Y, Cai J, Zhou T, et al. Improved long-term volume retention of stromal vascular fraction gel grafting with enhanced angiogenesis and adipogenesis. Plast Reconstr Surg 2018;141(5):676e–86e.
13. Wang J, Liao Y, Xia J, et al. Mechanical micronization of lipoaspirates for the treatment of hypertrophic scars. Stem Cell Res Ther 2019;10(1):42.
14. Sun M, He Y, Zhou T, et al. Adipose extracellular matrix/stromal vascular fraction gel secretes angiogenic factors and enhances skin wound healing in a murine model. Biomed Res Int 2017;2017:1–11.
15. Song YH, Shon SH, Shan M, et al. Adipose-derived stem cells increase angiogenesis through matrix metalloproteinase-dependent collagen remodeling. Integr Biol (Camb) 2016;8(2):205–15.

Fat Grafting for Facial Contouring (Temporal Region and Midface)

Yun Xie, MD*, Ru-Lin Huang, MD, PhD, Wenjin Wang, MD, PhD, Chen Cheng, MD, Qingfeng Li, MD, PhD*

KEYWORDS

- Facial contouring • Fat graft • Midface • Temporal hollowing • Fat compartment

KEY POINTS

- Targeted restoration of the facial fat compartments allows for safe, reproducible, and effective outcomes of facial contouring.
- The authors advocate grafting fat tissue first into the deep plane (deep facial fat compartments) and then the superficial plane (superficial fat compartments), the medial part and then lateral part, and the upper side and then lower side.
- Better volume augmentation is based on more living fat graft transfer provided; thus, the authors use the 3L3M technique to get more living fat granules to fill the soft tissue.

 Video content accompanies this article at http://www.plasticsurgery.theclinics.com.

INTRODUCTION

Facial volume loss in both bony and soft tissues results in hollowness and skin ptosis, which leads to concave facial contour, a deepened nasolabial fold, and midcheek groove, conveying an old and gaunt appearance. Autologous fat grafting is a well-accepted technique for soft tissue augmentation and has been advocated for facial contouring and body shape remodeling. There is no consensus in the literature, however, regarding the fat grafting technique, including the entry site for the cannula and the plane for fat placement. Historically, various fat grafting techniques have been developed and applied in clinical conditions and yield promising results, such as structure fat grafting (Coleman technique),[1] the 3M3L technique,[2] cell-assisted lipotransfer,[3] and nanofat grafting.[4] These techniques focus mainly, however, on the methodological aspects of fat harvesting, refining, and grafting skills in general.

Clinical observation and patient feedback reveal that long-term outcomes of fat grafting are diverse in different recipient sites, especially in the temporal region, one of the subunits with the lowest satisfaction rate after facial fat grafting. The authors believe the diversity of long-term outcomes of fat grafting is a result of different anatomic characteristics in different recipient sites that may directly influence grafted fat survival, neurovascular injury incidence, and fat tissue retention.

Based on these considerations and anatomic studies in the temporal region,[5] midface,[6] and hand,[7] the authors developed a concept of targeted fat grafting technique, which advocates targeted restoration of physiologic distribution and volume of fat compartments using anatomically

Disclosure Statement: The authors have nothing to disclose.
Shanghai Ninth People's Hospital, Shanghai Jiao Tong University School of Medicine, 19th Floor, Building 1, 639 Zhizaoju Road, Shanghai 200011, P.R. China
* Corresponding authors.
E-mail addresses: amiyayun@qq.com (Y.X.); dr.liqingfeng@yahoo.com (Q.L.)

Clin Plastic Surg 47 (2020) 81–89
https://doi.org/10.1016/j.cps.2019.08.008
0094-1298/20/© 2019 The Authors. Published by Elsevier Inc. This is an open access article under the CC BY-NC-ND license (http://creativecommons.org/licenses/by-nc-nd/4.0/).

adequate cannula entry sites and injection planes. The authors' previous clinical studies have demonstrated effective and safety profiles in facial contouring,[6] temporal hollowing augmentation,[5,8] and hand rejuvenation[7] and suggested more applications in other regions.

PREOPERATIVE EVALUATION AND SPECIAL CONSIDERATIONS

Each patient should be evaluated for general medical conditions in addition to some special preoperative evaluations, listed as follows:

1. Multiangles of standard photos—frontal, lateral, 45° lateral, 90° lateral, head up and head down, and some special angles—that can fully display the defect of face should be taken before operation. The photos can be printed to show patients where to fill and how thick they need to fill.
2. Three-dimensional (3-D) laser scan and 3-D volumetric analysis can be used to evaluate the symmetriy of the 2 sides of the face. The facial models are analyzed with corresponding analyzing software to quantify the volume discrepancy before graft, determining the quantity of the fat to inject.
3. For some pathologic soft tissue defects, such as radiation damage, scleroderma, and so forth, the skin may not have enough elasticity and be very tight or thin. The authors ask patient to stretch the skin for approximately 1 month to 3 months with small vacuum instruments or other tools to improve the recipient space.
4. CT scans may be used for Romberg disease patients at their first visit to make sure the atrophy degree of bone, muscle, fat tissue, and the occluding relation of their teeth.

The authors propose communicating well with each patient before operation for good compliance. Fat graft absorption is inevitable for every patient, especially during the first 3 months. To reach the final satisfactory results, patients may have injections 2 times to 3 times, with each time needing a 3-month to 6-month interval.

SURGICAL PROCEDURE

See Video 1. Before liposuction, the authors usually ask patients where the fattest part of their body is and for which part they most want to decrease the fat volume. Elderly women usually have fatty belly where abundant fat is easy to be suctioned. For young patients who do not have bigger belly, the authors prefer to get fat from their bilateral gluteal groove, which may have benefit for them to lift the most protruding point of gluteal and elongate the leg.

The second reason for harvesting fat from lower body position is because α-2 receptors located in diet-resistant areas such as the lateral thighs buttocks, and abdomen. The following are the procedure of 3L3M fat graft technique.

1. Fat graft harvest: the total fat volume the authors use is no more than 100 mL for facial contouring purposes; thus, the authors prefer harvesting fat 'Manually' or 'syringe suction'. The composition of tumescent anesthetic fluid is 0.08% lidocaine plus 1:500,000 epinephrine. After injecting tumescent for several minutes, the authors use a 20-mL syringe for hand liposuction. The authors keep 5 mL of air in the syringe before drawing back the Plunger pod and fixing it with a clamp or clip to create less negative pressure. The slower and gentler suction causes less oil from harvest fat. The authors may choose suction cannula with multiple side holes to do effective suction; the diameter of the side hole is chosen depending on the purpose of filling. For example, if volume augmentation and injecting to a deep layer are needed, a relatively larger hole, such as 2 mm to 3 mm, may be chosen. If injecting superficial layer or performing some subtle injection, the authors prefer smaller side holes to do suction.
2. Fat graft process: after acquiring fat, the authors use saline to wash away lidocaine, epinephrine, cell debris, and red blood cells. Lidocaine and epinephrine, which contain the tumescent, are reported to reduce the viability of adipocytes. Then, the authors stand the syringe with fat and saline for a while, until the lowest part of liquid looks relatively clear, which means there are fewer small adipocytes suspension in the liquid part. Thin patients may have more fibers than fat patients. Fibers in the harvested fat are cut into pieces before low-speed centrifugation. The fat samples are centrifuged at low speed, less than 100 g, for 2 minutes to 3 minutes. After centrifuge, the lowest liquid part is ejected out and then a 3-way or 2-way pipe connected to the 20-mL syringe to transfer the middle layer of fat into a 2-mL or 1-mL syringe. The top layer of oil is left in the syringe and used to lubricated inject cannula. The whole procedure is controlled at 25°C within 30 minutes to 60 minutes.
3. Recipient site preparation: Good design for patients should be done before surgery. 3-D

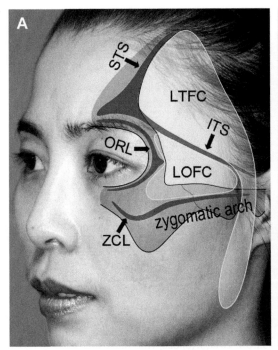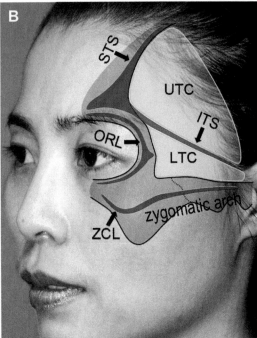

Fig. 1. Surface projection of fat compartments (*A*) and septum compartments (*B*) in the temporal region as demonstrated on a 37-year-old female patient. ITS, inferior temporal septum; LOFC, lateral orbital fat compartment; LTC, lower temporal compartment; LTFC, lateral temporal cheek fat compartmentORL, orbital retaining ligament; STS, superior temporal septum; UTC, upper temporal compartment; ZCL, zygomatic cutaneous ligament. (*From* Huang RL, Xie Y, Wang W, et al. Anatomical study of temporal fat compartments and its clinical application for temporal fat grafting. Aesthet Surg J. 2017;37(8):858; with permission.)

simulation or photos can help both surgeon and patients to make a decision. Make sure the recipient site is not injected with any other fillers, such as hyaluronic acid, collagen, and so on) or not use any enzyme to dissolve the fillers within 6 months. Make sure the skin has no infection (such as infectious acne) or ulceration, and the skin should have good elasticity to strut enough room for fat graft (**Figs. 1–6**).

Temporal hollowing augmentation can use the targeted fat grafting technique.Before fat grafting, the temporal hollowing region is marked by 4 borders:

1. Superiorly, the superior temporal line
2. Anteriorly, the lateral orbital rim
3. Inferiorly, the superior border of the zygomatic arch
4. Laterally, the temporal hair line

A small incision is made at the medial side of the head at the junction of the hairline and the temporal line. An 18G, single-holed, blunt-tipped infiltration cannula is inserted directly into this entry site and advanced along the surface of the skull until it enters the loose areolar tissue layer. Within this

layer, the fat graft is placed into the upper temporal and the lower temporal compartments using a multiplane, multitunneling technique. The infiltration cannula is withdrawn from the space under the superficial temporal fascia and advanced into the subcutaneous fat layer in the temporal region. In this plane, the fat should be precisely grafted to the lateral temporal cheek fat and the lateral orbital fat compartments to correct the irregularities of the skin caused by the deep plane injection. To form a round and convex facial contour, the infiltration cannula also may be inserted into the subcutaneous fat layer in the forehead to adjust the contour between the temporal and forehead regions.

Midface Fat Graft

The recommend incision is presented as following. A paraoral commissure incision was made on the lip mucosa 1 mm to 2 mm adjacent to the oral commissure to avoid any unwanted scar formation. An injection cannula was placed beneath the oral mucosa, in the muscle, or subcutaneously in the first injection point to ensure accurate placement of fat in different layers in subsequent

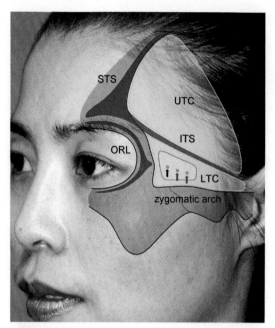

Fig. 2. Surface projection of the zone of caution as demonstrated on a 37-year-old female patient. The zone of caution is located in the lower temporal compartment at its anterior half, where the sentinel vein and branches of the middle temporal vessels perforate the temporal fascia and travel in the subcutaneous tissue layer (see arrows). ITS, inferior temporal septum; LTC, lower temporal compartment; ORL, orbital retaining ligament; UTC, upper temporal compartment; STS, superior temporal septum. (*From* Huang RL, Xie Y, Wang W, et al. Anatomical study of temporal fat compartments and its clinical application for temporal fat grafting. Aesthet Surg J. 2017;37(8):859; with permission.)

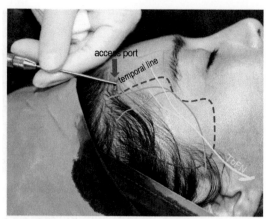

Fig. 3. The cannula entry site for temporal augmentation using fat grafting as demonstrated on a 37-year-old female patient. The entry site was placed medially to the junction of hairline and temporal line in an area that is relatively free of neurovascular structures. SV, sentinel vein; TbFN, temporal branch of the facial nerve. (*From* Huang RL, Xie Y, Wang W, et al. Anatomical study of temporal fat compartments and its clinical application for temporal fat grafting. Aesthet Surg J. 2017;37(8):860; with permission.)

procedures. The second choice of incision is making a punch following the nasal labial fold with a 16G needle and then placing a cannula, with a diameter smaller than 1.2 mm, that will not cause scarring.

The recommend injection technique is presented as followings. An 18G cannula connected to a 1-mL syringe was accurately placed beneath the lip mucosa or subcutaneously in the very beginning as required in subsequent procedures. When autologous fat was placed in the deep fat compartment, it was placed in the medial part of the deep medial cheek fat compartment by advancing the cannula between the mucosa and the orbicularis oris muscle. The root of the canine tooth was used as a bony marker to approach the medial part of the deep medial cheek fat compartment. The lateral part of the deep medial cheek fat compartment was approached by advancing the cannula in the same layer with the guidance of the first molar tooth and was

advanced close to the maxilla. The medial part of the suborbicularis orbital fat compartment was also approached by advancing the cannula in this trajectory in a line, connecting the first molar and the lateral limbus of the ipsilateral cornea. Special attention was paid to avoid advancing the cannula too close to the maxilla when the cannula was around the level of the nasal ala. From this incision, the cannula was directed laterally to the superior part of the buccal fat pad from the superoanterior quadrant of the medial wall of the buccal fat pad by advancing the cannula close to the maxilla.

For augmentation of the middle and lateral cheek fat compartments, the fat was placed by directing the cannula to the lower one-third of the masseteric ligament where the fibrous structure is weak. Alternatively, another incision in the sideburn was used to avoid any unwanted injury to the blood vessels or nerves in the masseteric ligament (See **Figs. 5** and **6**).

Case Demonstrations

Case 1

A 46-year-old female patient with severe deep temporal hollowness of both temples underwent 2 autologous fat grafting procedures for targeted restoration of temporal fat compartments (**Fig. 7**). In the first procedure, 20.0 mL of autologous fat was injected in the right temple and 18.0 mL on the left side; 3 months after the first fat grafting procedure, the patient underwent the second fat

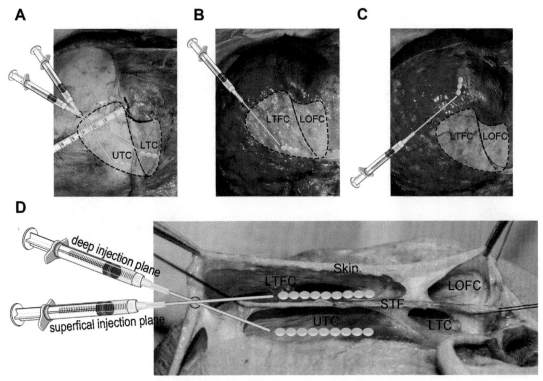

Fig. 4. Illustration demonstrating targeted fat grafting for temporal hollowing augmentation as demonstrated on a 72-year-old female cadaver. In this technique, the cannula entry is located medial to the junction of hairline and temporal line. The fat tissue is injected into the deep injection plane (*A*) in the loose areolar tissue layer (UTC and LTC), to restore the majority of volumetric loss, followed by an injection into the superficial injection plane (*B*) in the subcutaneous tissue layer (LFFC and LOFC), to achieve a smooth and round facial contour, and the transition zone (*C*) in the subcutaneous tissue layer of the frontal region, to achieve a smooth and round facial contour. (*D*) Illustration demonstrating the relationship of the superficial injection plane and the deep injection plane. LOFC, lateral orbital fat compartment; LTC, lower temporal compartment; LTFC, lateral temporal cheek fat compartment; STF, superficial temporal fascia; UTC, upper temporal compartment. (*From* Huang RL, Xie Y, Wang W, et al. Anatomical study of temporal fat compartments and its clinical application for temporal fat grafting. Aesthet Surg J. 2017;37(8):861; with permission.)

grafting procedure; 12.0 mL of fat was injected in each temple. At 12 months after the second fat grafting procedure, she presented only mild temporal hollowness in both temples.

Case 2

A 46-year-old female patient with moderate temporal hollowness of both temples underwent 1 autologous fat grafting procedure (**Fig. 8**); 18 mL of fat was grafted in each temple. Eighteen months after the fat grafting procedure, the patient appeared to have no hollowness in either temple.

Case 3

A 49-year-old female patient with temporal hollowness, obvious tear trough, and nasolabial folds of both sides underwent 1 autologous fat grafting procedure (**Fig. 9**). A total of 32 mL of fat was grafted in temporal region and midface. Twelve months after the fat grafting procedure, the patient

appeared to have no hollowness in either temple. The volume of midface was augmented.

POSTOPERATIVE CARE

Immediately after the procedure, a compression dressing was applied to the area for 5 days to 7 days. For patients who were not satisfied with the augmentation outcome, a second surgical procedure was performed 3 months to 6 months after the initial procedure to improve the contour.

EXPECTED OUTCOME AND MANAGEMENT OF COMPLICATIONS

After the fat grafting procedure using the targeted fat compartment volume restoration technique, the curvilinear line on the temporal region and midface became smoother and less concave. A pleasing result of an elevated anterior projection

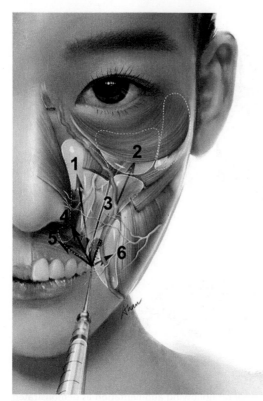

Fig. 5. Trajectory and sequence for deep fat compartment filtration. For fat placement in the deep cheek fat compartments, a specific sequence of fat placement is recommended: 1, medial part of the deep medial cheek fat compartment; 2, medial part of the suborbicularis oculi fat compartment; 3, lateral part of the deep medial cheek fat compartment; 4, lateral part of the nasal base; 5, upper lip in the submucosa layer; and 6, superior part of the buccal fat pad. (*Courtesy of* Zhou Shuyang.)

of the temporal region and midface was obvious. Complication was rare in the authors' case series. Minor complications, such as chronic edema, headache, and skin irregularity, were observed but fully recovered without treatment. Overcorrection was the most frequent reported major complication and was treated by liposuction. No infection, calcification, fibrosis, and fat embolism were reported in the authors' case series.

REVISION OR SUBSEQUENT PROCEDURES

Considering the resorption of fat graft, the second surgery usually is done after 3 months to 6 months. Most patients may have only a 1-time injection. Only a few of them have fat graft 3 or more times.

DISCUSSION

Anatomic and clinical studies have shown targeted restoration of the volume of facial fat

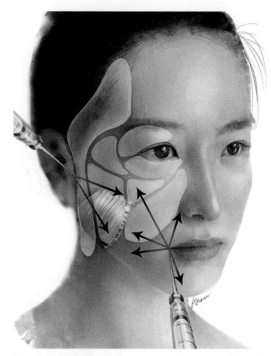

Fig. 6. Trajectory and sequence for superficial fat compartment infiltration through a paraoral commissure incision and an intraearlobe incision. The following sequence is recommended. First, direct the cannula laterally to approximately 1 cm lateral to the oral commissure, and turn upward toward the most prominent point of the zygoma and inject fat along the trajectory while withdrawing the cannula to create the upper half of the lateral border of the golden triangle (medial cheek fat compartment and nasolabial fat compartment). Second, direct the cannula laterally to approximately 1 cm lateral to the oral commissure and turn upward toward the mental tubercle and inject fat along the trajectory while withdrawing the cannula to create the lower half of the lateral border of the golden triangle. Third, direct the cannula to the nasolabial fat compartment and the medial cheek fat compartment medial and lateral to the lateral border of the golden triangle to create a smooth transition. Fourth, direct the cannula deep and along the nasolabial fold when necessary. For augmentation of the middle and lateral cheek fat compartments, another incision in the sideburn could be used as a complement to avoid any unwanted injury to the blood vessels or nerves in the masseteric ligament. (*Courtesy of* Zhou Shuyang.)

compartments by fat grafting not only restores the volume of facial fat compartments to a physiologic level and rebuilds a natural and youthful face but also avoids severe complications. Clinically, the 'temporal hollowing region' is different from a precise anatomic term, temporal fossa, and outlined by the superior temporal line, the

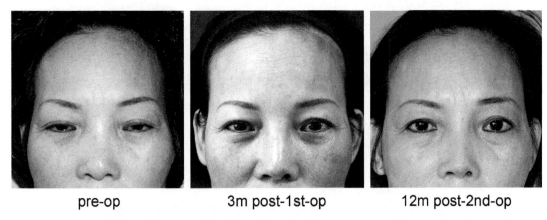

pre-op   3m post-1st-op   12m post-2nd-op

Fig. 7. Case 1: preoperative and postoperative photographs after fat grafting in the temple region. Right, pre-operation; middle, 3 months post-1st-operation; right, 12 months post-2nd-operation.

temporal hairline, the zygomatic arch, and the lateral orbital rim. In this region, 4 separated fat compartments overlap in 2 planes: the lateral temporal cheek fat compartments and lateral orbital fat compartments, located in the superficial plane, and the upper temporal compartments and lower temporal compartments, located in the deep plane. Several important neurovascular structures pass through these fat compartments, including the perforators of the middle temporal vein, the sentinel vein, the frontal branch of the superficial temporal artery, and the temporal branch of the facial nerve.[9] Therefore, the authors advocate that the fat tissue should be placed into the 4 temporal fat compartments through a unique entry site, which is located at the medial side of the intersection of the hairline and the temporal line.

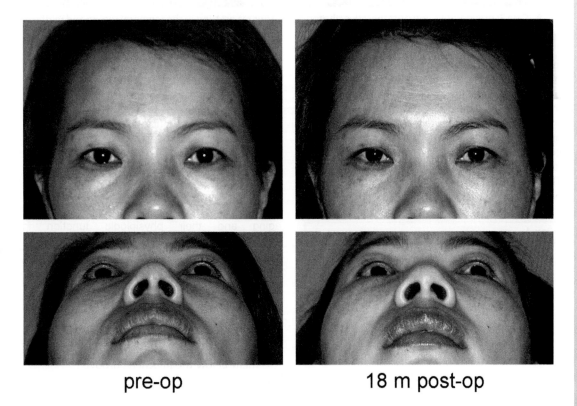

pre-op   18 m post-op

Fig. 8. Case 2: preoperative and postoperative photographs after fat grafting in the temporal region. Pre-op, pre-operation; 18 m post-op, 18 months post-operations.

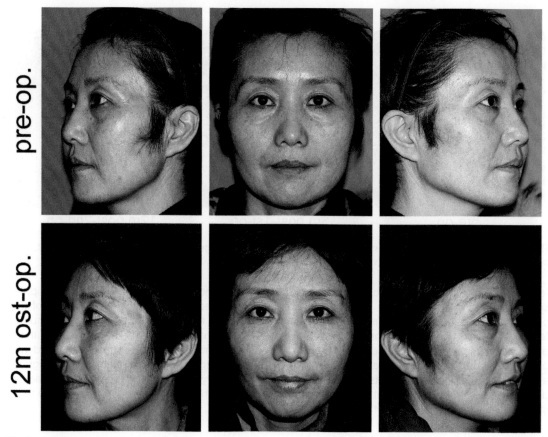

pre-op.

12m ost-op.

Fig. 9. Case 3: preoperative and postoperative photographs after fat grafting in the temporal region and midface.

In midface, the fat compartments are divided into superficial fat compartments (the superficial plane) and deep fat compartments (the deep plane). The deep fat compartments include the medial and lateral suborbicularis oculi fat compartments, the deep medial fat compartment, and the buccal fat compartment. These deep fat compartments support the fullness of the malar fat pad and play a major role in a youthful face. The superficial fat compartments include the nasolabial fat compartment, the cheek fat compartments, and the inferior orbital fat compartment.[10] The authors' strategy for midface fat grafting is designed with the aim of fat placement in a multiplane and compartment-specific manner to achieve a state close to the physiologic fat distribution of a youthful face. Taking the advantages of hidden location and accessibility to different layers, the paraoral commissure incision is advocated for grafting fat tissue to the superficial fat compartments and the deep fat compartments in midface. Considering the changes of the deep and superficial fat compartments caused by aging and their physiologic function in

---

Box 1
Recommended injection sequence of fat placement in the deep cheek fat compartments

1. Medial part of the deep medial cheek fat compartment
2. Medial part of the suborbicularis oculi fat compartment
3. Lateral part of the deep medial cheek fat compartment
4. Lateral part of the nasal base
5. Upper lip in the submucosa layer
6. Superior part of the buccal fat pad

Box 2
Recommended injection sequence of fat placement in the superficial fat compartments

1. Superior half of the medial cheek fat compartment below the lid-cheek groove
2. Superior part of the nasolabial fat compartment below the midcheek groove
3. Superior part of the nasolabial fat compartment below the tear trough
4. Below the nasolabial fold when necessary

constructing facial contour, a deep to superficial injection sequence is suggested. The recommended sequence of fat injection is shown in **Boxes 1** and **2**.

SUMMARY

Based on the authors' anatomic studies and clinical applications, the authors believe that compartment-based fat grafting is a safe and effective procedure for facial contouring for temporal region and midface.

ACKNOWLEDGMENTS

This work was supported by Project supported by the Funds for International Cooperation and Exchange of the National Natural Science Foundation of China (No: 81620108019); Natural Science Foundation of Shanghai (No: 17ZR1416500); Clinical Research Program of 9th People's Hospital (No: JYLJ004).

SUPPLEMENTARY DATA

Supplementary data related to this article can be found online at https://doi.org/10.1016/j.cps.2019.08.008.

REFERENCES

1. Coleman SR. Facial augmentation with structural fat grafting. Clin Plast Surg 2006;33(4):567–77.

2. Xie Y, Li Q, Zheng D, et al. Correction of hemifacial atrophy with autologous fat transplantation. Ann Plast Surg 2007;59(6):645–53.

3. Yoshimura K, Sato K, Aoi N, et al. Cell-assisted lipotransfer for facial lipoatrophy: efficacy of clinical use of adipose-derived stem cells. Dermatol Surg 2008; 34(9):1178–85.

4. Tonnard P, Verpaele A, Peeters G, et al. Nanofat grafting: basic research and clinical applications. Plast Reconstr Surg 2013;132(4):1017–26.

5. Huang RL, Xie Y, Wang W, et al. Anatomical study of temporal fat compartments and its clinical application for temporal fat grafting. Aesthet Surg J 2017; 37(8):855–62.

6. Wang W, Xie Y, Huang RL, et al. Facial contouring by targeted restoration of facial fat compartment volume: the midface. Plast Reconstr Surg 2017; 139(3):563–72.

7. Zhou J, Xie Y, Wang WJ, et al. Hand rejuvenation by targeted volume restoration of the dorsal fat compartments. Aesthet Surg J 2017;38(1):92–100.

8. Huang RL, Xie Y, Wang W, et al. Long-term outcomes of temporal hollowing augmentation by targeted volume restoration of fat compartments in Chinese adults. JAMA Facial Plast Surg 2018;20(5):387–93.

9. Sadick NS, Dorizas AS, Krueger N, et al. The facial adipose system: its role in facial aging and approaches to volume restoration. Dermatol Surg 2015;41(Suppl 1):S333–9.

10. Rohrich RJ, Pessa JE. The fat compartments of the face: anatomy and clinical implications for cosmetic surgery. Plast Reconstr Surg 2007;119(7):2219–27 [discussion: 2228–31].

Fat Grafting for Facial Contouring (Nose and Chin)

Tsai-Ming Lin, MD, PhD[a,b,*], Shu-Hung Huang, MD, PhD[b],
Yun-Nan Lin, MD[b,c], Su-Shin Lee, MD[b], Yur-Ren Kuo, MD, PhD[b],
Sin-Daw Lin, MD[b], Hidenobu Takahashi, MD[d]

KEYWORDS

• Facial contouring • Nose • Chin • Profiloplasty • Microautologous fat transplantation (MAFT)

KEY POINTS

• Microautologous fat transplantation (MAFT) has been postulated by the primary author, who have demonstrated its efficacy using the MAFT-GUN.
• The indispensability of MAFT in facial applications has been shown for sunken upper eyelid, temple and forehead recontouring, primary augmentation rhinoplasty, and gummy smile correction.
• The technique for Asian profiloplasty, using MAFT on the nasal dorsum and chin areas, has shown a favorable aesthetic result.

 Video content accompanies this article at http://www.plasticsurgery.theclinics.com.

INTRODUCTION

In 1963, Dr Landazuri was the first surgeon to use the term "profiloplasty," defined as rhinoplasty plus mentoplasty.[1] Asians often look to enhance the appearance of the nasal dorsum and chin profile due to certain ethnic deficiencies. Various nasal and chin implants have been adopted for this purpose. However, the results seemed unsatisfactory and potential morbidities were often bothersome. In past decades, fillers have garnered attention, despite complications and other concerns such allergy, necessity of repeat injection, and the cost-effectiveness.

Fat grafting was first described by Neuber in 1893[2] and continues to be performed frequently because of the ease of fat harvest, abundance of graft material, and the lack of transplant rejection. However, fat survival and retention rates are

Disclosure Statement: Dr T.-M. Lin owns the patent rights to the MAFT-GUN and is a scientific adviser for DermatoPlastica Beauty Co., the manufacturer of the MAFT-GUN device. None of the other authors have any financial disclosures or conflicts of interest.
Authorship: T.-M. Lin: First author and corresponding author with contribution to the surgical operation, data analysis, and interpretation. Y.-N. Lin, S.-H. Huang, S.S. Lee, Y.R. Kuo, S.D. Lin: Contributed to the data interpretation and analysis. H. Takahashi: Contributed to surgical operation, compiled the DVD, and created the animation.
^a Charming Institute of Aesthetic and Regenerative Surgery (CIARS), 2F.-1, No. 172, Ziqiang 2nd Road, Qianjin District, Kaohsiung City 801, Taiwan; ^b Division of Plastic Surgery, Department of Surgery, Kaohsiung Medical University Hospital, No. 100, Tzyou 1st Road, Kaohsiung City 807, Taiwan; ^c Division of Plastic Surgery, Department of Surgery, Kaohsiung Municipal Hsiao-Kang Hospital, Kaohsiung City, Taiwan; ^d Department of Surgery, Kaohsiung Medical University Hospital, No. 100, Tzyou 1st Road, Kaohsiung City 807, Taiwan, Taiwan
* Corresponding author. Charming Institute of Aesthetic and Regenerative Surgery (CIARS), 2F.-1, No. 172, Ziqiang 2nd Road, Qianjin District, Kaohsiung City 801, Taiwan.
E-mail address: k79157@gmail.com
Twitter: @TsaiMingLinMD (T.-M.L.)

Clin Plastic Surg 47 (2020) 91–98
https://doi.org/10.1016/j.cps.2019.08.009

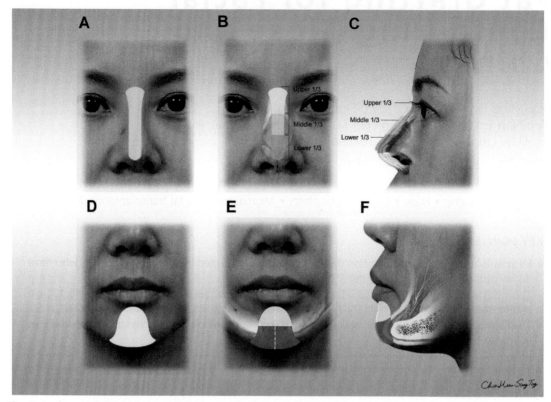

Fig. 1. In the nasal dorsum, the recipient area for fat transfer was drawn in the shape of an I (width, 6–8 mm) from the nasal tip to a point approximately 15 mm above the intercanthalline (*A*) with a fan-shaped cephalic end. This pattern was further divided into upper, middle, and lower zones (*B*). The fat parcels were transplanted in 3 layers (ie, from the deep areolar plane to the vascular/fibromuscular plane to the subcutaneous areolar plane) (*C*).[17] In the chin area, a bell shape was designed centrally from the margin of chin lower border to 5 mm above the mentolabial sulcus (*D*) further symmetrically divided into upper/lower, right/left portions. (*E*) Anatomic multiple-layer (deep: supraperiosteum, middle: periosteum to mentalis muscle/intermentalis muscle, superficial: mentalis muscle to skin) transplantation[18] was performed in chin area according to surgical planning. (*E and F, light brown*) For those who wish to reduce the sharpness of the mentolabial sulcus, MAFT was deployed in multiple layers from oral mucosa to sulcus skin (*E and F, yellow*). (*Courtesy of* Chia-Hsiu Chien and Siang-Ting Ciou.)

unpredictable, and complications such as abscesses, cysts, nodulation, and neurovascular injury may occur.[3]

Microautologous fat transplantation (MAFT) has been postulated by Lin and colleagues,[4] and its efficacy has been demonstrated using the innovative instrument, MAFT-GUN to illustrate the indispensability in clinical applications for facial and body contouring and rejuvenation.[5–13] In this article, the authors further demonstrate the technique for Asian profiloplasty of the nasal dorsum and chin areas to achieve favorable aesthetic appearance.

PREOPERATIVE EVALUATION AND SPECIAL CONSIDERATIONS

Preoperative evaluation included previous operative history and existing sequelae due to any filler injection. The best candidates for MAFT in these areas are patients without history of surgery (synthetic implant or autologous/allogenic cartilage or bone graft) or filler injections. Nevertheless, MAFT might be considered in selected cases due to unavoidable previous procedures.

Preoperative markings were made with the patient seated. In the nasal dorsum, the recipient area for fat transfer was drawn in the shape of an I (width, 6–8 mm) from the nasal tip to a point approximately 15 mm above the intercanthal line (**Fig. 1**A) with a fan-shaped cephalic end. This pattern was further divided into upper, middle, and lower zones (**Fig. 1**B). In the chin area, a bell shape was designed centrally from the margin of the chin to 5 mm above the mentolabial sulcus (**Fig. 1**D) that was further symmetrically divided into upper/lower, right/left portions (**Fig. 1**E). The recipient areas were multiple layers from deep, middle to superficial layers (**Fig. 1**C, F).

SURGICAL PROCEDURE

All patients received total intravenous anesthesia before fat grafting. Appropriate local anesthesia was applied at donor and recipient inserting sites with 0.3 to 0.5 mL of 2% lidocaine HCl with epinephrine (1:50,000). Lipoaspirates were harvested from the lower abdomen or inner thigh where the adipocyte viability was greater.[14] The donor site was infiltrated with a tumescent solution (10 mL of 2% lidocaine [20 mg/mL]: 30 mL of Ringer lactate solution: 0.2 mL of epinephrine [1:1000]). Approximately 10 to 15 minutes after infiltration, fat was harvested from the donor site with a blunt-tip cannula (diameter, 2.5 or 3.0 mm; ≥1 holes sized 1 mm × 2 mm). The lipoaspirate volume was approximately equal to the volume of the tumescent solution to ensure that fat constituted a major proportion of the lipoaspirate. To minimize damage to the lipoaspirate, the plunger of a 10-mL syringe connected to a liposuction cannula was withdrawn to approximately 2 to 3 mL to maintain a negative pressure of 270 to 330 mm Hg.[15] Lipoaspirates were processed and purified by centrifugation at 3000 rpm (approximately 1200 g) for 3 minutes as described by Coleman.[16] This procedure minimized graft contamination due to environmental exposure and manual manipulation. Centrifugation facilitated separation of the lipoaspirate into layers. The top layer contained oil from ruptured fat cells; the middle layer contained purified fat; and the bottom layer contained blood, cellular debris, and fluid. The purified fat was carefully transferred into a 1-mL Luer-slip syringe using a transducer. The syringe containing purified fat was loaded into a MAFT-GUN (**Fig. 2**) and connected to an 18-gauge, blunt-tip cannula. The device was set by adjusting a dial to deliver fat parcels of 0.0067 mL (ie, 1/150 mL) to 0.0083 mL (ie, 1/120 mL) with each trigger deployment (see **Fig. 2**). A puncture incision was made on the nasal tip/bilateral mouth angles with a no. 11 scalpel blade (see **Fig. 1**B, E) as an insertion point.

Fat Grafting Injection

Microautologous fat transplantation to the nasal dorsum
The fat transplantation procedure to the nasal dorsum was performed by pulling the trigger while withdrawing the MAFT-GUN. Meticulously, the parcels were transplanted in 3 layers of the nasal dorsum from the deepest to the most superficial layers (ie, from the deep areolar plane to the

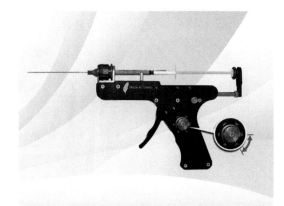

Fig. 2. The purified fat is transferred to a 1-mL syringe and loaded in a MAFT-GUN (Dermato Plastica Beauty Co., Ltd., Kaohsiung, Taiwan). The volume of a single delivered fat parcel is set between 1/150 mL (0.0067 mL) to 1/120 mL (0.0083) by turning the 6-graded volume dial to 150 or 120.

vascular/fibromuscular plane to the subcutaneous areolar plane) (see **Fig. 1**C).[8,17] During MAFT, downward traction was applied to successive zones of the nose with the surgeon's nondominant hand. First, traction was placed on the middle third of the nose while grafting the upper third. Next, traction was placed on the lower third of the nose (ie, the nasal tip) while grafting the middle third. Fat was transferred to the nasal tip last.[8] The nasal dorsum is roughly divided by three (upper-, middle- and lower-third) as figure. The volume of fat grafting to be transplanted on nasal dorsum was roughly distributed on each third. However, the upper third was approximately 40-50% of the total volume. The insertion wound was subsequently closed with 1 suture (6-0, nonabsorbable) (Videos 1 and 2).

Microautologous fat transplantation to the chin
Anatomic multiple-layer (deep: supraperiosteal, middle: periosteal to mentalis muscle/intermentalis muscle, superficial: mentalis muscle to skin) transplantation[18] was performed in the chin area according to surgical planning (see **Fig. 1**E, light brown). For those who wished to reduce the sharpness of the mentolabial sulcus, MAFT was particularly emphasized to blend this sulcus for a pleasing obtuse appearance (see **Fig. 1**E, yellow). Although in this sulcus, the multiple-layer transplantation was also applied from oral mucosa to skin. The average volume in this sulcus area was 1.0 to 2.0 mL (see **Fig. 1**E, yellow) and the volume of the chin augmentation was 2.0 to 4.0 mL (see **Fig. 1**E, light brown). The bilateral insertions were closed with 6-0 nonabsorbable sutures (Videos 3 and 4).

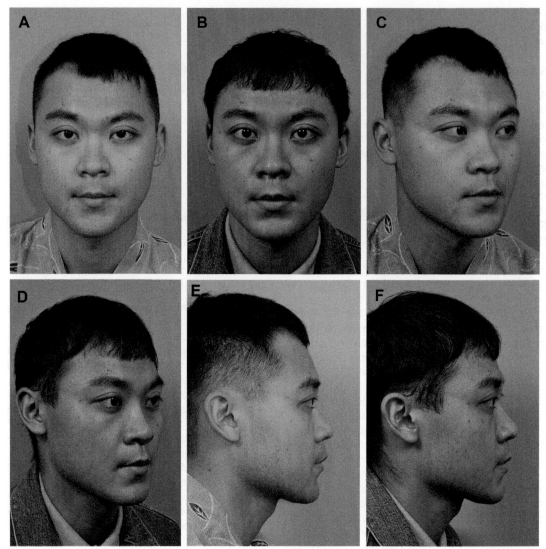

Fig. 3. A 26-year-old man presented for augmentation rhinoplasty with fat grafting to increase the height and length of his nose (A, C, E). MAFT was performed to place a 3.5-mL fat graft (1.5, 1.0, and 1.0 mL in the upper, middle, and lower thirds of the nasal dorsum, respectively). One year after a single MAFT session (B, D, F), the fullness over nasal dorsum was shown with the height and length maintained.

POSTOPERATIVE CARE

Massage was avoided postoperatively in the recipient area. The donor area was dressed with compressive garments and the recipient with adhesive paper tape to alleviate swelling. Routine postoperative care, oral antibiotics, and nonsteroidal antiinflammatory drugs were administered for 3 days or as needed. The suture placed at the insertion site was removed 2 to 3 days postoperatively, and the sutures placed at the donor site were removed 1 week postoperatively. Gentle lymphatic drain massage was suggested 7 days after surgery to relieve swelling. All patients received routine follow-up at an outpatient clinic at 1, 3, 6 months and even longer postoperatively. Photographs were taken at each visit for comparisons over time.

EXPECTED OUTCOME AND MANAGEMENT OF COMPLICATIONS

About 80% of patients in the authors' series (more than 500 cases, recontouring for nasal dorsum/ chin or combined) for profiloplasty by MAFT technique were satisfied with a single procedure. No infections, cyst formations, nodulations, irregularities, or any severe complications were reported.

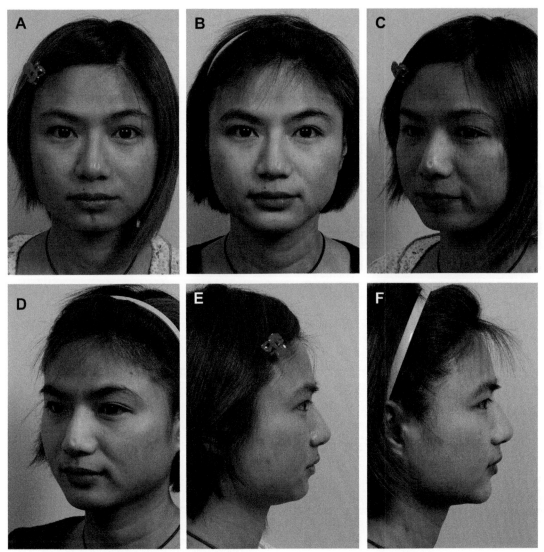

Fig. 4. A 34-year-old woman presented for recontouring of her chin that had showed central depression (cleft chin) since her teenage years (*A, C*). A just-healed carbuncle was noted with erythematous change on the day of surgery. She underwent one session of MAFT over the chin area designed as **Fig. 1**E, F (*light brown*). A total of 4 mL of fat was grafted symmetrically over the chin. Eleven months after the MAFT session, the results were stable and the chin contouring were well maintained (*B, D*). The retrusion of her chin was well contoured showing the effectiveness of the MAFT in profile views (preoperative *E*, postoperatively *F*).

REVISION OR SUBSEQUENT PROCEDURES

Touchup MAFT might be performed 4 to 6 months after the first procedure for those who requested further enhancement of the contouring.

CASE DEMONSTRATIONS

Case 1. See **Fig. 3**.
Case 2. See **Fig. 4**.
Case 3. See **Fig. 5**.
Case 4. See **Fig. 6**.

DISCUSSION

Despite the fact that fat grafting has become popular in the past decade, several unresolved issues exist for fat grafting procedures. Particularly, patient dissatisfaction often occurs because of unpredictable absorption rates and potential morbidities such as visible nodulation and fibrosis.[3] There remains a lack of evidence regarding long-term outcomes. Lin and colleagues[4] demonstrated the clinical feasibility and indispensability of MAFT for facial recontouring

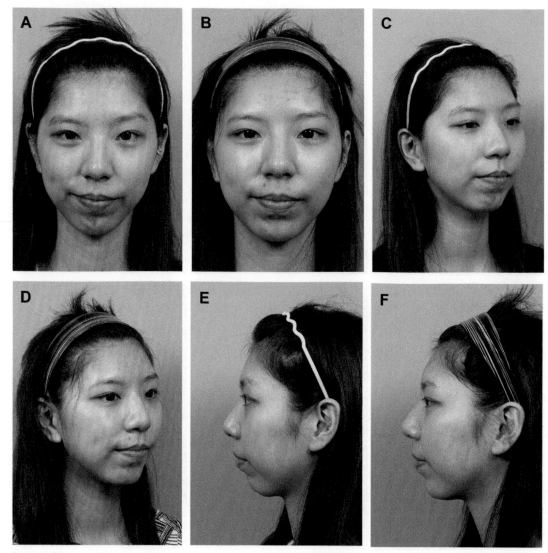

Fig. 5. A 26-year-old woman presented for recontouring of her chin and nose (*A, C, E*). She underwent MAFT procedure with a total of 3 mL of fat grafted over her nasal dorsum (1 mL for each one-third portion). For recontouring her retrusion chin with mentalis muscle strain, 2 mL of fat graft in the mentolabial sulcus area (see **Fig. 1**E, F, *yellow*) and 5 mL of fat graft over chin area (see **Fig. 1**E, F, *light brown*) were evenly transplanted. One year after MAFT, the pleasing facial contouring of her nose and chin was effectively illustrated (*B, D, F*). The improved mentalis strain appearance was maintained and with proportional height/length of nose and chin contour.

and rejuvenation of the sunken upper eyelids,[5,6] nasal dorsums,[8] temples,[9] and foreheads.[10] They also proposed a new strategy for combined augmentation of the nasolabial groove, ergotrid, and upper lip for the treatment of gummy smile, illustrating an easy, reliable approach for facial contouring.[12]

The concept of MAFT, as proposed by Lin and colleagues in 2007,[4,19] emphasized that the volume of each delivered parcel should be less than 1/100 mL (<0.01 mL) to avoid potential fat grafting morbidities.[3] The patented MAFT-GUN[19] provides surgeons with a tool to control the parcel volume

and therefore substantially avoid central necrosis and its associated complications. The long-term results specifically demonstrated accurate and consistent control of the fat parcels (1/60, 1/90, 1/120, 1/150, 1/180, and 1/240 mL) by avoiding occasional dislodgement of larger parcels that result in central necrosis and subsequent nodularity and skin irregularity over time.[5–13]

There are numerous strategies for facial contouring for the nose and chin and each has its individual indications and potential complications. Nevertheless, no single procedure fulfills all the requests from all patients. With application of MAFT, the

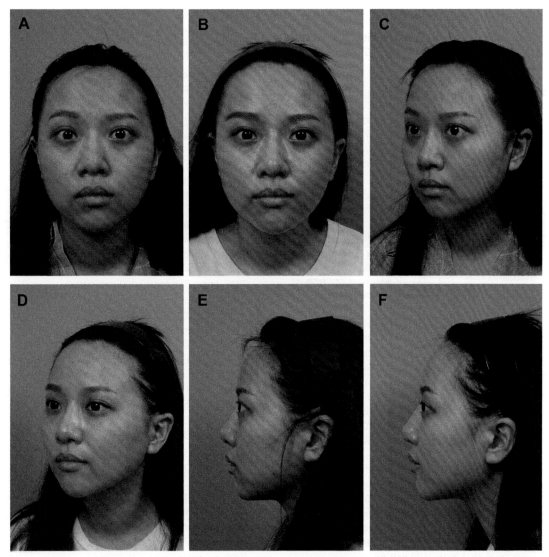

Fig. 6. A 24-year-old woman presented for facial contouring on her nose and chin (*A, C, E*). The MAFT procedure for augmenting the height and length of her nose with advancement of her chin was performed. A total of 3 mL of fat was grafted over her nasal dorsum (each 1.0 mL in the upper, middle, and lower thirds of the nasal dorsum, respectively). For chin advancement and elongation, 2 mL of fat graft in the mentolabial sulcus area (see **Fig. 1**E, F, *yellow*) and 4 mL of fat graft over chin area (see **Fig. 1**E, F, *light brown*) were evenly transplanted. One year after MAFT (*B, D, F*), the results were stable and effective. The facial contouring was well reconstructed and the sharpness of mentolabial sulcus was improved.

traditional morbidities after fat grafting are decreased with promising long-term results. Furthermore, the rejuvenating effects of skin texture are also noted (see **Figs. 4** and **5**), further demonstrating the feasibility of fat grafting for facial contouring of the nose and chin.

SUMMARY

In search for a better profiloplasty strategy in Asians, there are many strategies with individual indications. Nevertheless, there seems to be no single way to fulfill all the goals. By avoiding the potential complications of fat grafting, MAFT provides an innovative breakthrough strategy in precise delivering of small fat parcels. The authors presented a simple, reliable, and consistent procedure developed based on MAFT for profiloplasty. Favorable outcomes with sustainable long-term effectiveness were obtained, further confirming that the MAFT technique is an alternative for facial contouring in the nose and chin.

SUPPLEMENTARY DATA

Supplementary data related to this article can be found online at https://doi.org/10.1016/j.cps.2019.08.009.

REFERENCES

1. Landazuri HF. Profiloplasty (rhinoplasty and mentoplasty). Ann ChirPlast 1963;8:191–7 [in French].
2. Neuber GA. Fettransplantation. Chir Kongr Verhandl Deutsche Gesellschaft fur Chir 1893;22:66.
3. Khawaja HA, Hernández-Pérez E. Fat transfer review: controversies, complications, their prevention, and treatment. Int J Cosmet Surg Aesthetic Dermatol 2002;4(2):131–8.
4. Lin TM, Lin SD, Lai CS. The treatment of nasolabial fold with free fat graft: preliminary concept of Micro-Autologous Fat Transplantation (MAFT). Paper presented at: The 2nd Academic Congress of Taiwan Cosmetic Association Taipei. Taiwan, May 7, 2007.
5. Lin TM, Lin TY, Chou CK, et al. Application of micro-autologous fat transplantation in the correction of sunken upper eyelid. Plast Reconstr Surg Glob Open 2014;2(11):e259.
6. Lin TM, Lin TY, Huang YH, et al. Fat grafting for re-contouring sunken upper eyelids with multiple folds in Asians-novel mechanism for neoformation of double eyelid crease. Ann Plast Surg 2016;76(4):371–5.
7. Lin TM. Total facial rejuvenation with micro-autologous fat transplantation (MAFT). In: Pu LLQ, Chen YR, Li QF, et al, editors. Aesthetic Plastic Surgery in Asians: Principles and Techniques. 1st edition. St. Louis (MO): CRC Press; 2015. p. 127–46.
8. Kao WP, Lin YN, Lin TY, et al. Microautologous fat transplantation for primary augmentation rhinoplasty: long-term monitoring of 198 Asian patients. Aesthe Surg J 2016;36(6):648–56.
9. Lee SS, Huang YH, Lin TY, et al. Long-term outcome of microautologous fat transplantation to correct temporal depression. J Craniofac Surg 2017;28(3):629–34.
10. Chou CK, Lee SS, Lin TY, et al. Micro-autologous fat transplantation (MAFT) for forehead volumizing and contouring. Aesthetic Plast Surg 2017;41(4):845–55.
11. Lin YN, Huang SH, Lin TY, et al. Micro-autologous fat transplantation for rejuvenation of the dorsal surface of the aging hand. J Plast Reconstr Aesthet Surg 2018;71(4):573–84.
12. Huang SH, Huang YH, Lin YN, et al. Micro-autologous fat transplantation for treating a gummy smile. Aesthet Surg J 2018;38(9):925–37.
13. Huang SH, Lin YN, Lee SS, et al. Three simple steps for refining transcutaneous lower blepharoplasty for aging eyelids: the indispensability of micro-autologous fat transplantation. Aesthet Surg J 2019. https://doi.org/10.1093/asj/sjz005.
14. Geissler PJ1, Davis K, Roostaeian J, et al. Improving fat transfer viability: the role of aging, body mass index, and harvest site. Plast Reconstr Surg 2014;134(2):227–32.
15. Chou CK, Lin TM, Chiu CH, et al. Influential factors in autologous fat transplantation - focusing on the lumen size of injection needle and the injecting volume. J IPRAS 2013;9:25–7.
16. Coleman SR. Structural fat grafting. Aesthet Surg J 1998;18(5):386–8.
17. Wu WT. The Oriental nose: an anatomical basis for surgery. Ann Acad Med Singapore 1992;21(2):176–89.
18. Kim BJ, Lim JW, Park JH, et al. Dual plane augmentation genioplasty using gore-tex chin implants. Arch Craniofac Surg 2014;15(2):82–8.
19. United States Patent, Patent No.: US 7,632,251 B2. 2009.

Fat Grafting for Facial Contouring Using Mechanically Stromal Vascular Fraction–Enriched Lipotransfer

Natale Ferreira Gontijo-de-Amorim, PhD[a,b,c,d,e,*], Luiz Charles-de-Sá, PhD[c,d,e,f], Gino Rigotti, MD[c,d,g]

KEYWORDS

- Stem cells • Adipose-derived stem cells • Stem cell-enriched lipotransfer • Fat graft
- Fat transplantation • Stromal vascular fraction

KEY POINTS

- The preferred donor site for lipotransfer in face should be the lower abdomen. The fat is harvested with syringe, creating a light negative pressure by slowly withdrawing the plunger in a manual gradual manner.
- Part of the aspirated fat is allowed to set for decantation and washing with saline. Other part is processed in a centrifuge for mechanical isolation of the stromal vascular fraction (SVF) to prepare the mechanically SVF-enriched fat.
- The fat is injected using a multichannel technique, retrogradely in each movement until achieving volume augmentation, avoiding overcorrection.
- The postoperative absorption index of the injected enriched fat is low compared with traditional fat grafting.
- The mechanically SFV-enriched lipotransfer technique does not use enzymatic process, does not involve any expensive machinery or devices, and is easily reproducible.

INTRODUCTION

Fat is an ideal tissue as an autologous substitute with which tissue deficiencies can be treated . It is available in easily accessible subcutaneous depots but also can be molded to reconstruct defects. Unfortunately, despite more than 100 years of clinical use, the clinical longevity of the fat graft is highly variable, is operator-dependent, and has a high ratio of absorption; in particular, the volume of large grafts decreases significantly over time.[1] The presumed mechanisms of tissue loss seem primarily insufficient vascularity, cell death, and other mechanisms, such as mechanical disruption of cells, lipid-induced membrane damage, and apoptosis.[2]

Nowadays, it is known that adipose tissue is rich in regenerative cells, such as stem cells, more than bone marrow. Adipose-derived stem cells (ADSCs) were identified by Zuk and colleagues[3] in 2001. These investigators defined the ADSC characteristics by their ability to differentiate into several mesenchymal lineages. ADSCs can be isolated from the stromal vascular fraction (SVF)

Disclosure Statement: The authors have nothing to disclose.
[a] Pontifical Catholic University of Rio de Janeiro (PUC - Rio) and Carlos Chagas Post-graduation Institute (Pitanguy Institute), Rio de Janeiro, Brazil; [b] Verona University - Italy, Verona, Italy; [c] ASPS; [d] ISPRES; [e] FILACP; [f] Training and Research State University Hospital of Rio de Janeiro - Brazil (UERJ), Rio de Janeiro, Brazil; [g] Regenerative Surgery Unit, San Francesco Clinic, Verona, Italy
* Corresponding author. Rua Visconde de Pirajá, 351 salas 1211 e 1212, Ipanema, Rio de Janeiro Cep: 22410-003, Brazil.
E-mail address: natalefga@yahoo.com.br

Clin Plastic Surg 47 (2020) 99–109
https://doi.org/10.1016/j.cps.2019.08.012
0094-1298/20/© 2019 Elsevier Inc. All rights reserved.

through enzymatic process and culturing on plastic because, unlike the other cell types in SVF, they adhere to plastic. The recognition that fat contains multipotent stem cells that can be harvested through liposuction without altering their viability has driven further examination into the potential uses of fat and its ADSCs.[4,5] The aspirated fat has approximately half the number of the adipose mesenchymal stem cells found in excision whole fat.[6] The relative deficiency of ADSC yield may be one of the reasons for long-term atrophy of transplanted aspirated adipose tissue. The clinical potential of supplementing fat grafts with more ADSCs has been reported as a novel method of autologous tissue transfer, termed cell-assisted lipotransfer.[7,8] The potential benefits of ADSCs are promising, because they have several advantages over fat grafting alone.

In this article, the authors introduce a structural fat grafting procedure[9] associated with a new model of cell-assisted lipotransfer technique in the management of volumetric deficit of the face in pathologies, such as Romberg syndrome and trauma sequelae, and also in the aged face, to determine an easy and reproducible method that can yield higher concentrations of preserved adipocytes and ADSCs that could guarantee long-lasting results. The enrichment of fat presented in this article is based on another study that compared the effects of the 3 most common fat processing techniques used in plastic surgery (decantation, washing, and centrifugation) on the viability and number of cellular components of aspirated adipose tissue, determining a method that can yield higher concentrations of viable adipocytes and mesenchymal stem cells.[10,11] The whole surgical lipotransfer was performed bedside, and enzymatic digestion process was not used to prepare the enriched fat, called by the authors mechanically SVF-enriched (MeSe) lipotransfer technique.

PREOPERATIVE EVALUATION AND SPECIAL CONSIDERATIONS

For the management of volumetric deficit of the face, in cases of facial deformities, such as Romberg syndrome and trauma sequelae, the preoperative work-up included laboratory studies, blood test, cardiac examination, photography, and sliced 3-dimensional (3-D) tomography. The amount of fat to be implanted was assessed based on degree volume deficit. In the cases of Romberg syndrome and trauma sequelae, the parameter was the contralateral hemiface that was normal. After obtaining successful results in these unilateral deformities, the mechanically

SVF-enriched lipotransfer technique was applied in the treatment of the aged face.

All patients were clearly informed of the benefits, risks, operative complications, and postoperative care and gave their informed consent to the intervention. Furthermore, all patients were submitted to the surgery in hospital environment.

The patients consented under approved guidelines set for human clinical trials by the Brazilian investigation ethics committee board (protocol no. 28063) and the Brazilian Clinical Trials Registry (Rebec. UTN: U1111–1145–3081).

SURGICAL PROCEDURE
Donor Site Selection

When the lipotransfer is executed in the face, donor sites are selected considering the easy accessibility in the supine position, avoiding changes in the position of the patient during the surgery. In general, the authors prefer the lower abdomen as a donor area. In addition to avoiding the change of decubitus, a higher concentration of ADSCs was found in the lower abdomen.[12]

Fat Harvesting

After antiseptic cleaning of the skin with chlorhexidine, the fat was collected from the lower abdomen using the super wet technique. A solution containing normal saline and 0.5% lidocaine with 1:500,000 of epinephrine was injected through a 22-gauge spinal needle before aspiration. It was infiltrated into the area of liposuction at a ratio of 1 mL of solution per milliliter of aspirated tissue. The mean quantity of 200 mL of harvested fat was aspirated using blunt cannulas of 3 mm in diameter and 20 cm in length (tip model 3B, Richter, São Paulo, Brazil) attached to a 10-mL Luer lock syringe, creating a light negative pressure by slowly withdrawing the plunger in a manual gradual manner.

Fat Purification and Mechanical Stromal Vascular Fraction Enrichment of the Fat

After collection, the adipose tissue was separated into 2 groups. Half of the syringes were allowed to set for decantation under the action of gravity for 15 minutes. After this, the inferior layer, composed mostly of blood, was thrown out and the remaining fat was washed with saline to remove blood and cell elements and left to stand; 3 washes yielded a layer of saline and a supernatant predominantly comprising bright yellow adipocytes. This procedure was done using the same 10-mL Luer lock syringe used during fat harvesting, and the piston was never removed from the harvesting syringe during washing to avoid tissue exposure to air. The other half of the volume of the aspirated fat was processed in a centrifuge for mechanical isolation of the SVF. This half of the collected fat that was placed in capped 10-mL syringes was put in a centrifuge (IEC Medilite Microcentrifuge, Thermo-electron Corporation, Byron Medical, USA) and spun at 3000 rpm for 3 minutes, equivalent to 1286 g. In the final centrifugation process, 4 basic layers were observed macroscopically. The fourth layer, called the pellet, at the bottom of the centri-fuged sample, corresponds to the SVF, a pool of regenerative cells that was separated by mechan-ical dissociation without enzymatic process (**Fig. 1**).

To prepare the mechanically SVF-enriched fat, each 10-mL syringe with washed fat was enriched with the pellet of 1 centrifuge sample and gently mixed, after connecting to fill Luer lock syringes via syringe adapter (female Luer lock adapter).

One syringe of 10 mL of washed fat and 1 pellet of the centrifuge sample collected from each pa-tient were sent to the laboratory and analyzed by the same group of biotechnicians, less than 24 hours after the collection. After discarding the superior and inferior layers of washed lipoaspirate, the middle layer, which is routinely used for adi-pose tissue graft, was kept for analysis.

Implant Site of the Mechanically Stromal Vascular Fraction–Enriched Lipotransfer Technique

Preoperative markings were done in face, identi-fying the areas of volumetric deficit (**Fig. 2**). Su-praorbital, infraorbital, and mental nerve block was achieved with 1 mL to 2 mL of 2% lidocaine when under sedation and locoregional anesthesia.

Aimed at carrying out the fat implantation, small scalp incisions were made with an 18G needle and the mechanically SVF-enriched fat was injected into the target sites. The fat was injected using a 2-mm to 3-mm blunt-tipped Coleman cannula connected to syringe, using a multichannel tech-nique, retrogradely in each movement (**Fig. 3**). The amount of fat to be implanted was assessed based on degree volume deficit, avoiding overcor-rection and aiming at observing the degree of fat absorption. The parameter in the cases of Rom-berg syndrome and trauma sequelae was the contralateral hemiface that is healthy. Fat was homogeneously deposited in the subcutaneous level in multiple layers to achieve volume augmen-tation in these cases, always avoiding overcorrec-tion (**Fig. 4**).

In cases of an aged face, a solution of saline and 0.5% lidocaine with 1:200,000 epinephrine was

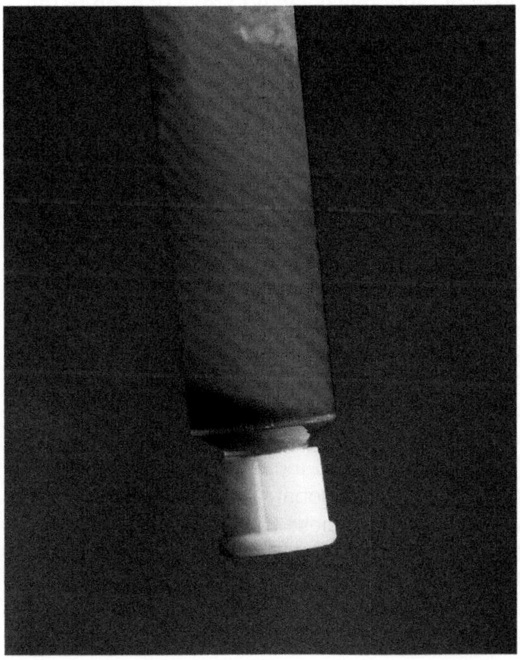

Fig. 1. The layer, called pellet, at the bottom of the centrifuged sample corresponds to the SVF, a pool of regenerative cells that was separated by mechanical dissociation without enzymatic process.

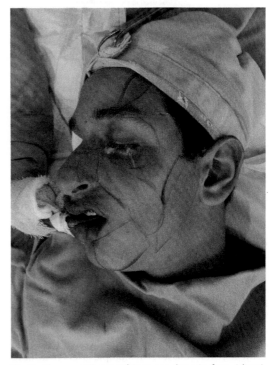

Fig. 2. Preoperative markings are done in face, identi-fying the areas of volumetric deficit.

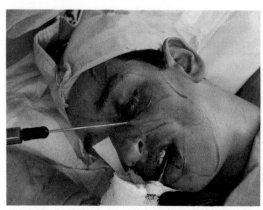

Fig. 3. The fat is injected using 2-mm to 3-mm blunt-tipped Coleman cannula connected to syringe, using a multichannel technique, retrogradely in each movement.

injected subcutaneously fanwise around the areas to be treated with lipofilling, because midface lift surgery was executed for the replacement of the malar fat pad,[13] prior to lipotransfer. In undermined areas of the midface, lipofilling was injected in the sub–superficial musculoaponeurotic system

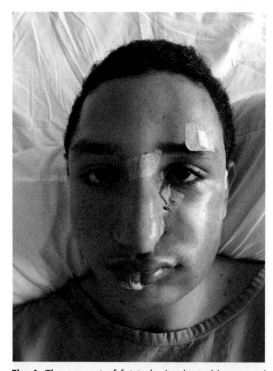

Fig. 4. The amount of fat to be implanted is assessed based on degree volume deficit. The parameter in the cases of Romberg syndrome is the contralateral hemiface that is healthy. Fat is homogeneously deposited in the subcutaneous level in multiple layers to achieve volume augmentation in these cases, avoiding overcorrection.

(SMAS) layer, at the same surgical time. In the intact areas, lipofilling was executed in subcutaneous layer.

The region of lipotransfer was gently massaged and the cannula access points were sutured with 6.0 nylon suture.

ADDITIONAL EVALUATIONS
Histologic Analysis of the Adipocytes

Lipoaspirate fragments of the washed sample were placed on paper filters and fixed in 10% formaldehyde in phosphate-buffered saline (PBS) at pH 7.4 for 24 hours to 48 hours at room temperature. After fixation, the tissues were dehydrated in graded ethanol, cleared in xylol, and embedded in paraffin at 60°C. Five-μm sections cut at 100-μm intervals on an American optical microtome were stained by hematoxylin and periodic acid–Schiff. Two sections of each sample were examined for architectural disruption, degeneration, or necrosis of the adipocytes, using a digital camera coupled to an image acquisition program (Q-Capture, Quantitative Image Corporation). Measurements were performed by 2 observers on blinded samples within adipocyte lobules, using Image Pro-Plus software (Media Cybernetics), and included cell count of only intact adipocytes per high-powered ($\times$ 200) field on 15 high-powered images of randomly selected areas of each paraffin section.

Obtaining Hematopoietic and Nonhematopoietic Cells by Mechanical Dissociation

Each sample was distributed into tubes containing ammonium–chloride–potassium buffer solution (1/1, vol/vol). The resulting mixture was shaken and maintained at 37°C for 15 minutes for red blood cell lysis. The cells were then separated from oil and other debris by centrifugation at 900 g for 15 minutes at room temperature. Next, they were washed with PBS containing 3% bovine serum albumin (PBS-BSA 3%) and incubated for 30 minutes at 4°C with monoclonal antibodies conjugated with fluorescent dies: CD14-PE, CD16-PE-Cy7, CD31-PE, CD34-PerCP-Cy5.5, and CD45-FITC (BD Biosciences, Franklin Lakes, New Jersey) and CD105-PE (R&D Systems, Minneapolis, Minnesota). After incubation, they were washed with PBS-BSA 3%. When necessary, the cell suspension was incubated at room temperature in the dark for 10 minutes with FACS Lysing Solution (BD Biosciences).

Flow Cytometry Analysis of the Adipose-Derived Mesenchymal Stem Cells of Washed Lipoaspirate and Pellet

The cells were then stained with propidium iodide (Sigma-Aldrich, St. Louis, Missouri) to assess their viability. Two populations of cells were distinguished: nonviable hematopoietic cells positive for CD45, CD14, and CD16, and viable ADSCs positive for CD105, CD90, CD73, CD146, and CD34 and negative for CD45. Subsequent analyses were performed using a FACSCanto (BD Biosciences) equipped with the software FACSDiva 4.0. Simultaneously, the obtained cells were quantified by Turk staining on a hematocytometer under a microscope. Then, the total cell number obtained from 1 g of suctioned adipose tissue processed from washed technique was calculated. Alternatively, pellets collected from the centrifuged samples were also subjected to the same protocol to obtain the relative and absolute number of stem cell population.

POSTOPERATIVE CARE

The grafted areas cannot be manipulated by vigorous massages or any direct trauma that could compromise fat graft survival.

EXPECTED OUTCOMES AND MANAGEMENT OF COMPLICATIONS

The clinical final results of mechanically SVF-enriched lipotransfer technique were assessed by observation, examination with palpation, and preoperative and postoperative photographs at least during the postoperative period of 1 year. In the cases of Romberg syndrome and trauma sequelae, the patients were also submitted to preoperative and postoperative 3-D tomography scan after 2 years of the surgery. The 3-D image done in the area submitted to the SVF-enriched lipotransfer showed the same tissue characteristics as those of the healthy contralateral side, without cyst, fibrosis, and calcifications (case 1). The quantity of SVF-enriched fat graft ranged between 10 mL and 100 mL, depending on volumetric deficit. The absorption index was minimal after at least 12 months during postoperative period (cases 1–3).

Histologic analysis of adipocytes and flow cytometry of mesenchymal cell population in the washed lipoaspirate and pellet samples were carried out (**Table 1**).

The morphology and quantity of adipocytes were analyzed in washed lipoaspirate sample, revealing a high number of intact adipocytes, with preservation of their initial morphology. After

Table 1
Quantitative representation of hematopoietic (CR45$^+$) and nonhematopoietic (CD45$^-$) cell fraction in washed lipoaspirate and pellet samples

	Washed Lipoaspirate	Pellet
CD45$^+$ = hematopoietic cells	2.5 ± 0.8	8.7 ± 1.3
CD45$^-$ CD31$^+$ = endothelial cell	4.7 ± 1.6	6.5 ± 2.0
CD45$^-$ CD34$^+$ = mesenchymal cell	4.2 ± 0.9	4.1 ± 1.9
CD45$^-$ CD106$^+$ CD90$^+$ CD73$^+$ CD105$^+$ = mesenchymal cell	4.3 ± 1.2	4.7 ± 1.6

The table represents the percentages of cell in each sample.

laboratory analysis of the pellet, it was found that this layer was rich in ADSCs (**Fig. 5**).

REVISION OR SUBSEQUENT PROCEDURES

The mechanically SFV-enriched lipotransfer technique demonstrated a low absorption index after at least 12 months of postoperative follow-up (cases 1–3), so a second section of lipotransfer was not requested by the patients.

It was also observed that the quality of the skin was improved in the areas that received the SVF-enriched lipotransfer (case 4).

CASE DEMONSTRATIONS
A 26-Year-Old Woman

See **Fig. 6**.

An 18-Year-Old Man

See **Fig. 7**.

A 58-Year-Old Woman

See **Fig. 8**.

A 48-Year-Old Woman

See **Fig. 9**.

DISCUSSION

The use of adipose tissue for effective treatment of facial and body enhancement and recontouring in patients presenting atrophy of soft tissues from aging and loss from congenital deformities and acquired pathologies has been shown attractive

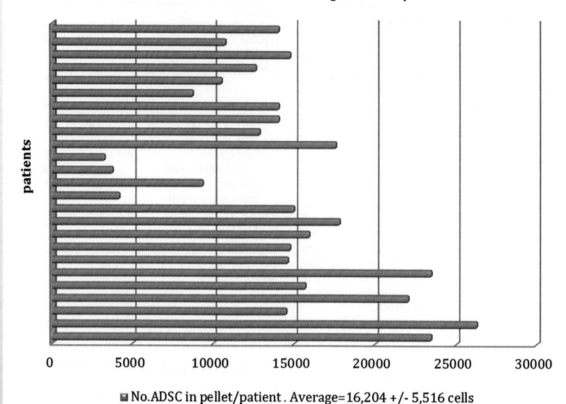

Fig. 5. Quantitative number of mesenchymal cell fraction in pellet samples by flow cytometry (CD105$^+$/CD90$^+$/CD73$^+$/CD146$^+$/CD14$^-$/CD45$^-$/CD34$^-$), representing the total number of mesenchymal cells and its average in 25 pellet/patient samples.

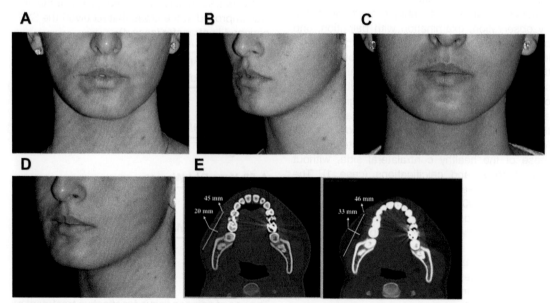

Fig. 6. Case 1: a 26-year-old woman with Romberg syndrome, preoperative (*A, B*) and 2 years postoperative (*C, D*). The 3-D tomography scan of preoperative period was compared with the 3-D CT, 2 years after the surgery using mechanically SVF-enriched lipotransfer technique, and showed the same tissue characteristics as those of the healthy contralateral side, without cyst, fibrosis, and calcifications (*E*). This patient experienced a volume decrease of 6% based on CT findings.

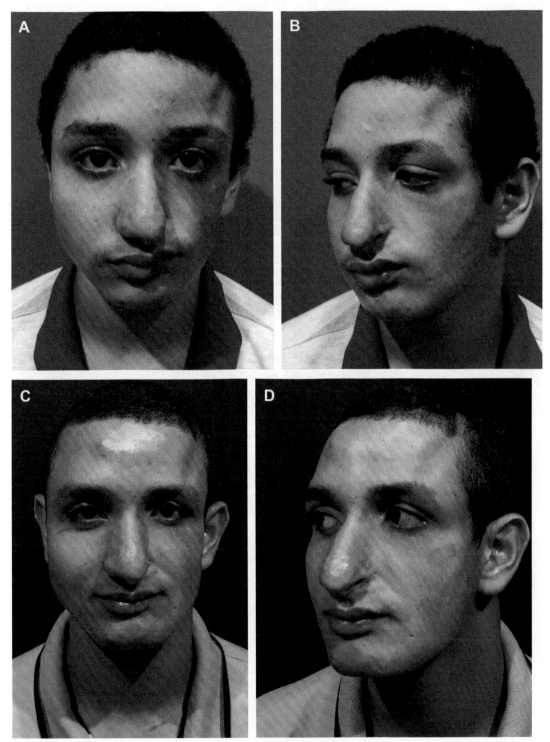

Fig. 7. Case 2: the patient, an 18-year-old man with Romberg syndrome (*A*, *B*), received mechanically SVF-enriched fat lipotransfer to the face (70 mL); after 5 years of follow-up (*C*, *D*), showed improvement after a single lipotransfer surgery, without overcorrection or requirement of reviews.

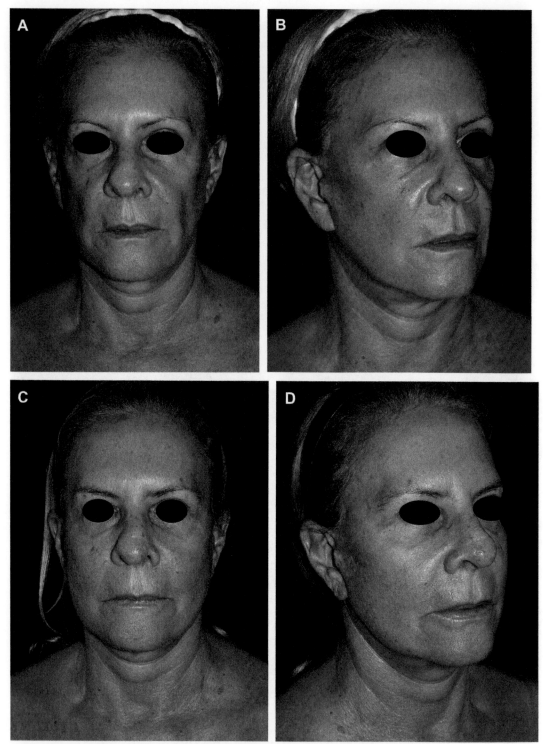

Fig. 8. Case 3: the patient, a 58-year-old woman, complained about an aged face and referred 2 face-lifts previously (*A*, *B*). Midface lift was executed for the replacement of the malar fat pad and SMAS, prior to lipotransfer. In undermined areas of the midface, lipotransfer was injected in the sub-SMAS layer and, in the intact areas, lipotransfer was executed in subcutaneous layer, at the same surgical time; 1 year postoperative period showed improvement of facial volumetry (*C*, *D*).

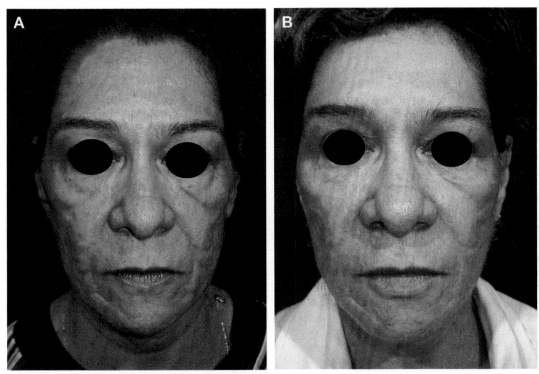

Fig. 9. Case 4: the patient, a 48-year-old woman, complained about aged face and acne sequelae (*A*) and blepharoplasty and SVF-enriched lipotransfer were indicated. It was observed that the quality of the skin was improved in the areas that received the SVF-enriched fat, as well as facial volumetry, after 2 years of follow-up (*B*).

because it is readily available, inexpensive, and host compatible and can be harvested easily and repeatedly as needed without worry of allergic or foreign-body reaction.[14] Unfortunately, in practice, fat transplantation often has unreliable long-term results because of absorption and volume loss. As a result, several different techniques of lipofilling have been developed in recent years.[15] Considering the variety of approaches, therefore, the ones using ADSCs seem most promising, termed cell-assisted lipotransfer.

In this study, the authors have proposed the use of washed lipoaspirate enriched with the SVF of the fat to produce the mechanically SVF-enriched lipotransfer technique, based on fewer red blood cells and white blood cells, extracellular free lipids, and less damaged tissue and debris, with higher structural stability of the adipocytes, such as their viability and high concentration of regenerative cells. On the other hand, this fat tissue processing preserves the cells of the SVF and growth factors owing to the fact that such factors are water-soluble.[10,11,16] Although 1 g of excised adipose tissue yielded nearly 5000 ADSCs, the lipoaspirate presented one-half of this quantity.[7] The mechanically SVF-enriched lipotransfer technique turns

ADSC-poor aspirated fat into ADSC-rich fat.[17] This cell-assisted strategy, by mechanical dissociation of the SVF, increased the number of ADSCs, on an average, more 1600 cells per milliliter in each 10-mL syringe (more 16,000 ADSCs in 10 mL of fat) (see **Fig. 5**). This fact can justify the authors' satisfactory results.

Beyond the previous fact explained, the preparation of the SVF-enriched fat using mechanical separation of the SVF in a proper layer by centrifugation is demonstrated in this article. The harvested cells were surrounded by a glycoprotein scaffold, including tissue factors that would be eliminated with digestion of the matrix, if treated with collagenase.[18] The loss of cell viability caused by the use of enzymes, such as collagenase, during cell harvesting and processing has already been described in several protocols of primary cell cultures. So the mechanical process is proposed as a preferable method for preservation of ADSC properties in samples.[19] Also, processes based on enzymatic digestion seemed less reproducible and expensive.[18]

Nowadays, one phenomenon, which was initially underestimated but whose importance has recently emerged, is the action of the stem cell niche, which seems stronger than that of the isolated stem cell.[20] The interaction between all cells, as an entity of action with cytokines and growth factors involved, is more important to fat survival than the isolation of a specific cell from the fat to after mixing it again in the fat. Adult or somatic stem cells generally have limited function without the niche, and the integration of stem cells into tissues is the basis for higher forms of life.[20] Treatment with mechanically SVF-enriched lipotransfer technique in the surgical room without any digestion of cells or expansion in vitro seems to be a method particularly suitable for the reconstruction of stem cell niches for other tissues. The interaction between the transferred regenerative cells and the host tissue in the stable condition is the important key to successful results. The ADSCs were used for the purpose of enhancing angiogenesis and reducing the absorption rate of fat grafts and postoperative atrophy. In addition, the structural fat grafting procedures associated with minimal manipulation and trauma of the lipoaspirate should be encouraged to reach predictable and long-lasting results.[17] Even more, the use of ADSC is a promising technique for rejuvenation of the human skin, as demonstrated in previous articles.[21,22]

SUMMARY

Structural fat grafting associated with cell-assisted lipotransfer technique in the management of volumetric deficit of the face demonstrated that the Mechanically SVF-enriched lipotransfer technique or MeSe lipotransfer technique maintains high cell viability. Prospective results proved that fat grafts processed by this technique are easily reproducible and have higher survival rate with volume maintenance of transplanted fat and normal tissue characteristics, without fibrosis, cysts, and calcifications. This method does not involve any expensive machinery, so has low cost. It is a safe and effective procedure, with all patients showing improvement after a single lipotransfer surgery, without overcorrection or requirement of reviews after at least 1 year of follow-up.

REFERENCES

1. Peer LA. Loss of weight and volume in human fat grafts. Plast Reconstr Surg 1950;5:217–30.
2. Brown SA, Levi B, Lequeux C, et al. Basic science review on adipose tissue for clinicians. Plast Reconstr Surg 2010;126:1936–46.
3. Zuk PA, Zhu M, Mizuno H, et al. Multilineage cells from human adipose tissue: implications for cell-based therapies. Tissue Eng 2001;7:211–28.
4. Rigotti G, Marchi A, Galiè M, et al. Clinical treatment of radiotherapy tissue damage by lipoaspirate transplant: a healing process mediated by adipose-derived adult stem cells. Plast Reconstr Surg 2007;119:1409–22.
5. Gir P, Oni G, Brown SA, et al. Human adipose stem cells: current clinical applications. Plast Reconstr Surg 2012;129:1277–90.
6. Matsumoto D, Stao K, Gonda K, et al. Cell-assited lipotransfer (CAL): supportive use of human ADSCs for soft tissue augmentation with lipoinjection. Tissue Eng 2006;12:3375–82.
7. Yoshimura K, Sato K, Aoi N, et al. Cell-assisted lipotransfer for facial lipoatrophy: efficacy of clinical use of ADSCs. Dermatol Surg 2008;34:1178–85.
8. Tiryaki T, Findikli N, Tiryaki D. Staged stem cell-enriched tissue (SET) injections for soft tissue augmentation in hostile recipient areas: a preliminary report. Aesthetic Plast Surg 2011;35:965–71.
9. Coleman SR. Facial recontouring with lipostructure. Clin Plast Surg 1997;24:347.
10. Conde-Green A, Gontijo de Amorim NF, Pitanguy I. Influence of decantation, washing and centrifugation on adipocyte and mesenchymal stem cell content of aspirated adipose tissue: a comparative study. J Plast Reconstr Aesthet Surg 2010;63:1375–81.
11. Condé-Green A, Baptista LS, Gontijo de Amorim NF, et al. Effects of centrifugation on cell composition and viability of aspirated adipose tissue processed for transplantation. Aesthet Surg J 2010;30(2):249–55.
12. Geissler PJ, Davis K, Roostaeian J, et al. Improving fat transfer viability: the role of aging, body mass index, and harvest site. Plast Reconstr Surg 2014;134:227–32.
13. Pitanguy I, Radwanski HN, Gontijo de Amorim NF. Treatment of the aging face using the "Round-lifting" technique. Aesthet Surg J 1999;19(3):216–22.
14. Pu LLQ, Coleman SR, Cui X, et al. Autologous fat grafts harvested and refined by the Coleman technique: a comparative study. Plast Reconstr Surg 2008;122:932–7.
15. Ross RJ, Ramin S, Mutimer KL, et al. Autologous fat grafting current state of the art and critical review. Ann Plast Surg 2013;00:01–6.
16. Zhu M, Cohen SR, Hicok KC, et al. Comparison of three different fat graft preparation methods: gravity separation, centrifugation and simultaneous washing with filtration in closed system. Plast Reconstr Surg 2013;131:873–80.
17. Gontijo-de-Amorim NF, Charles-de-Sá LA, Rigotti G. Mechanical supplementation with the stromal vascular fraction yields improved volume retention in facial lipotransfer: a 1-year comparative study. Aesthet Surg J 2017;37(9):975–85.
18. Rigotti G, Marqui A, Sabarbati A. Adipose-derived mesenchymal stem cells: past, present, and future. Aesthetic Plast Surg 2009;33:271–3.

19. Shah FS, Wu X, Dietrich M, et al. A non-enzymatic method for isolating human adipose tissue-derived stromal stem cells. Cytotherapy 2013;15:979–85.

20. Scadden DT. The stem-cell niche as an entity of action. Nature 2006;441(29):1075–9.

21. Charles-de-Sa L, Gontijo-de-Amorim NF, Takiya CM, et al. Antiaging treatment of the facial skin by fat graft and adipose-derived stem cells. Plast Reconstr Surg 2015;135(4):999–1009.

22. Rigotti G, Charles-de-Sá L, Gontijo-de-Amorim NF, et al. Expanded stem cells, stromal-vascular fraction, and platelet-rich plasma enriched fat: comparing results of different facial rejuvenation approaches in a clinical trial. Aesthet Surg J 2016; 36(3):261–70.

Fat Grafting for Pan-Facial Contouring in Asians
A Goal-Oriented Approach Based on the Facial Fat Compartments

Li Zhanqiang, MD

KEYWORDS

- Fat injection • Facial fat compartments • Facial contouring • Personal approach

KEY POINTS

- The author introduces a fat injection approach for facial contouring of young Asian women.
- This method is based on the theory of facial fat compartments, and goal is to distribute facial highlights and shadows needed by Asian women.
- The approach includes the choice of incision, level of injection, and quantity of injection needed in different parts, named as functional zones and transition zones.
- At the present time, this approach has achieved very stable and satisfactory results in the author's clinical practice.

 Video content accompanies this article at http://www.plasticsurgery.theclinics.com.

INTRODUCTION

Facial fat injection is a common procedure worldwide. It is widely used in facial rejuvenation, soft tissue augmentation, and other applications. However, the procedure is not considered to have consistent results and no single procedure is widely accepted. The fates of the injected fat grafts are also not certain.[1–4] Some authors argue that the fat should be injected into fat pad,[5] whereas others think it should be injected into the muscle.[6] Each option has its advantages and has produced good results, but none have earned the full confidence of the medical community.

The facial fat compartment theory supports a promising method. Drs Rohrich and Pessa have brought the concepts of fat deposition and smooth transition between compartments to plastic surgeons' attention.[7,8] The first author of the current work, who completed his fellowship in 2008 at UT Southwestern, learned a great deal about fat injection from these 2 researchers. After returning to China, the author gradually developed a personal pan-facial injection approach based on their findings. A classification method based on Asian aesthetic goals was here used to guide the deposition volume. Over the past 6 years, as more consistent results have been achieved, the approach was considered fully developed, and major revisions ceased. In this article, the details underlying this approach are presented and the results are reviewed.

PREOPERATIVE EVALUATION AND SPECIAL CONSIDERATIONS

All patients desired pan-facial fat injection to improve their facial contouring. All patients were female. Before surgery, I discuss with patients about the injection areas, possible

Disclosure Statement: The author has nothing to disclose.
Myoung Medical Cosmetic Hospital, Wangjing Xiyuan San Qu, Wangjing Street, Chaoyang District, Beijing 100102, China
E-mail address: leezhanqiang@hotmail.com

Clin Plastic Surg 47 (2020) 111–117
https://doi.org/10.1016/j.cps.2019.08.014

complications and considerations during recovery period. For some hesitant patients, I also choose to use 3-dimensional simulation to help them determine whether the effect after surgery is consistent with their expectations. I point out the location where the skin will be pierced. The planned harvested area of lateral thigh is also evaluated to estimate the amount of fat expected to be collected. Details of the design and manipulation process are detailed here and shown in the videos.

SURGICAL PROCEDURE
Planning and Preparation

First, the premaxilla zone, here called as the first functional zone, is marked. The expected height of this zone is matched to the virtue curve between zygomatic arch and nasal tip. Then the transition zones around this functional zone, such as the nasolabial groove and cheek depression, are noted. As described in the Fat Harvesting section, the expected height of eyebrows, here called the second functional zone, is balanced with the nasal tip and the chin (**Fig. 1**). The other zones are designated as transition zones, covering the areas from the functional zones to the hidden sites, such as hair-bearing areas. The borders between functional zones and transition zones are actually anatomic borders between fat compartments.

All the procedures are performed under general anesthesia. No tumescent techniques are used in fat harvesting, and no local anesthesia is administered to the recipient sites. The eyelids are closed with a 6-0 nylon suture before injection.

Fat Harvesting

The most common donor site is the lateral thigh, but occasionally the inner thigh or abdomen are also used. After the patient is prepared, a 50-mL syringe and sharp 3-mm cannula with multiple holes are used to harvest fat from the deep layer only. Normally, 80 to 100 mL of lipoaspirate is sufficient for pan-facial fat injection.

Fat Processing

The lipoaspirate is centrifuged at 2000 rpm for 3 minutes. The product has 3 layers. The uppermost layer and dark bottom layer are discarded. The central layer, a mixture of fat and blood plasma, is transferred into a 1-mL syringe for injection.

Fat Injection

A blunt, 1.5-mm cannula with a single side-hole is used for facial fat injection. Injection begins from the premaxillary area for contouring. For the first step, the cannula is placed through the mucosa of the gingival sulcus, normally with a finger press on the infraorbital rim for protection (**Fig. 2**). This injection layer is very deep, close to the surface of the bone. The plunger is pushed very softly as the syringe is retracted, leaving a well-proportioned 0.2 to 0.3 mL fat graft per line in the tissue. Then the cannula is pushed into the

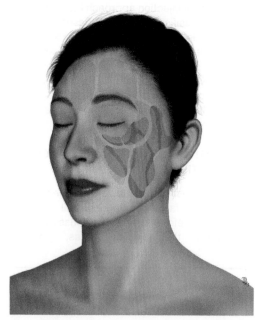 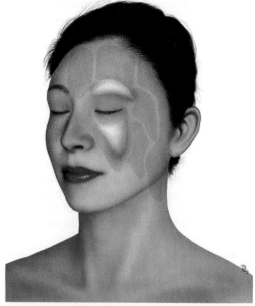

Fig. 1. (*Left*) Facial fat compartments. (*Right*) The premaxillary zone and eyebrow zone are classified as functional zones and other fat compartments as transition zones.

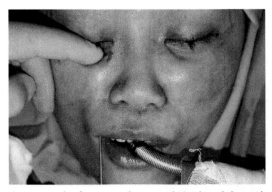

Fig. 2. For the first step, the cannula is placed through the mucosa of the gingival sulcus, normally with a finger pressed on the infraorbital rim for protection.

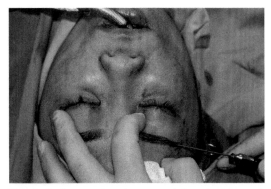

Fig. 4. Eyebrow, also the second function zone, is injected.

tissue just beside the previous line. This injection maneuver is repeated during the next retraction again until a fan-shaped area is completed. Then, with a fresh syringe, another layer is laid above the previous one, also in a fan shape. In this way, 3- to 6-mL grafts are placed, according to the height needed (Video 1).

The next injection point is through the mucosa in the nostril. This layer is more superficial, located within the subcutaneous layer, crossing the previous layer. The transition to the infraorbital rim was performed through this point with very tiny fat droplet (**Fig. 3**, Video 2).

Also through this point, 1- to 2-mL grafts are injected into the nasolabial groove, very deep, close to the surface of the bone surface, to soften the transition between the premaxillary area and upper lip (Video 3).

The next injection point is the tail of the eyebrow. A puncture is made in the skin with an 18G needle, then the fat injection cannula was placed through the subcutaneous layer. This sets the contour and height of the new eyebrow (**Fig. 4**). The new eyebrow's contouring

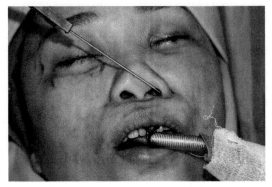

Fig. 3. Through the mucosa in the nostril, a superficial layer of premaxilla zone and deep layer of nasolabial groove are injected.

balance with the new radix, while at the peak of the forehead in the profile. More grafts are left in the medial part of the eyebrow and fewer in the lateral part. This contouring can bring a flat face forward rather than outward. During the injection, the left finger is pressed against the superior orbital fissure to protect the vessels from injury (Video 4).

The frontal and temporal areas are all accessed through this injection point. The frontal injection layer is subgalea layer and the temporal area is the subcutaneous layer. A half-circle injection in a fan-shaped pattern is centered around this small hole as a center, and a half-circle injection is made. All of the injected graft margin is hidden behind the hairline (Videos 5 and 6).

For cases requiring injection into the cheek area, an injection point just below the zygomatic arch is best. The aim of the injection is to soften the transition between the arch and the cheek. Here, a 1- to 2-mL subcutaneous injection is enough for that (Video 7).

Another injection point in the midline of the frontal hairline can also be used, cross-injecting with previous injection lines to make the forehead even. The injection must be made carefully in the glabella area, in line with the medial part of the eyebrow.

Finally, through the point at the eyebrow tail, a smooth transition is made between the first functional zone and the cheek (**Fig. 5**). After the middle of the face is brought forward by the premaxillary area injection, there is a shadow at the side of the deposited mass. The cannula is placed through this groove, carefully injecting a tiny drop as it is retracted. Sometimes there is also a groove between the temporal and cheek areas, just above the arch. This transition should be made smooth during this step (Video 8). The volume of fat placement in different areas are listed in **Table 1**.

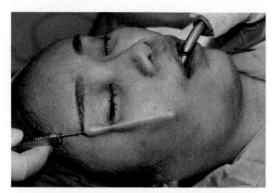

Fig. 5. Through the point at the eyebrow tail, a smooth transition is made between the first functional zone and the cheek.

POSTOPERATIVE CARE

Routine antibiotics are given for 3 days. No massage, hot or cold compress on the face, or diet is permitted after surgery for 3 months. The patient normally returns to social activity, with makeup, in 15 days. During the postoperative period, patients were followed to evaluate the results and record possible complications at months 1, 3, 6, 12, and 24. The results were clinically and photographically documented.

EXPECTED OUTCOME AND MANAGEMENT OF COMPLICATIONS

In the present study, 105 patients with a mean age of 25.8 years (range, 19–38 years) from 2009 to 2016 were enrolled. All the patients were followed for an average of 19.6 months (range, 6–47 months). The overall evaluation was performed by inspection, palpation, and photographic documentation. All patients were asked

Table 1
Volume of fat placement in different areas

Site (per Side)	Range (mL)	Average (mL)
Premaxilla	3–7	4.5
Nasolabial groove	1–2	1.5
Eyebrow	1–3	2.0
Temple	1–3	2.0
Frontal	15–30	21.4
Cheek	1–2	1.8
Transition between premaxilla and cheek	1–2	1.5
Chin	2–6	4.3
Mandibular	1–2	1.3

about their level of satisfaction 1 year after surgery simply asking for a yes or no answer to whether they were satisfied with the result. Out of the 105 patients, 101 answered yes (96.1%). The other 4 said no, giving the reason that they "could not accept the new face" or that there was "too much fat on the face." One of these unsatisfied patients underwent liposuction of the face 1 year after the first surgery, having 3 mL of fat removed. The other 3 patients declined the proposed additional refinements. No major complications such as infection, cysts, or edema were observed in any of these patients.

REVISIONS OR SUBSEQUENT PROCEDURES

In the author's series, 97 patients received only 1 procedure and 8 patients had a second procedure.

CASE DEMONSTRATIONS
Case 1

A 36-year-old woman underwent a single procedure with 2.5 years of follow-up. The procedure was combined with a costal cartilage rhinoplasty. Her weight before surgery was 47 kg and 49 kg at the last follow-up (**Fig. 6**).

Case 2

A 27-year-old woman underwent a single procedure with 2 years of follow-up. The procedure was combined with a costal cartilage rhinoplasty. Her weight before the surgery was 51 kg and 52 kg at the last follow-up. She is the patient shown in the video (**Fig. 7**).

Case 3

A 31-year-old woman underwent a single procedure with 1.5 years of follow-up. The procedure was combined with a rhinoplasty for her deviated nose. Her weight before surgery was 46 kg and 48 kg at the last follow-up (**Fig. 8**).

DISCUSSION

In traditional Asian culture, a beautiful female face should be round and full, with well-proportioned features and distribution of highlights and shadows. That ideal is the major reason for the increasing demand for facial fat injection in the first author's medical practice. In this cohort, the average age was much younger than in the studies run by Rohrich and Pessa.[9] This is partially because most of the author's patients were requesting rhinoplasty and facial contouring rather than rejuvenation. During the early years, the

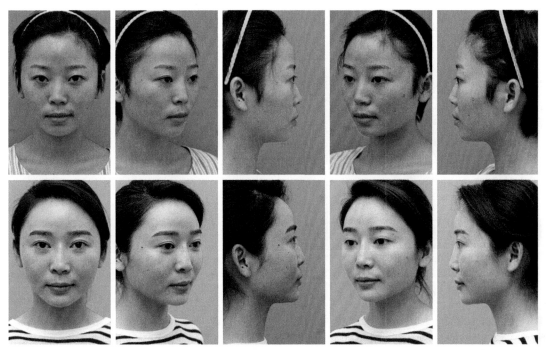

Fig. 6. Case 1. Preoperative (*upper*) and postoperative views (*lower*, 2.5 years postoperatively with fat injection).

author performed some fat injection principally to balance the new nose. As more and more patients reported satisfaction with the appearance of their whole faces, the author started to develop the approach described here to produce consistent results. The fat compartment theory is the principal basis for this approach. The clinical results

reported here provide evidence to support this theory.

These younger patients have tighter skin. During injection into the subcutaneous layer, distinct borders between compartments can be observed from the surface with the naked eye. These borders cannot be smoothed by pressing on the

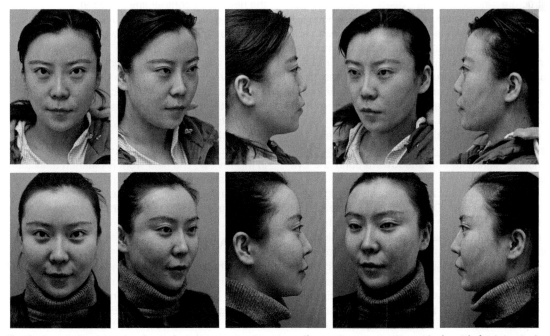

Fig. 7. Case 2. Preoperative (*upper*) and postoperative views (*lower*, 2 years postoperatively with fat injection).

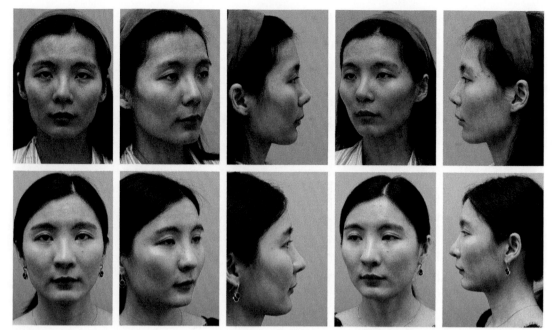

Fig. 8. Case 3. Preoperative (*upper*) and postoperative views (*lower*, 1.5 years postoperatively with fat injection).

injection sites with the fingers. However, digital manipulation can be used to flatten any minor irregularity within a single compartment.

The compartment distribution model distinguishes functional zones from transitional zones. It is a goal-oriented classification method based on anatomic findings. The current findings are consistent with Dr Rohrich's assertion that the most important compartment for reshape of facial structure including the deep medial cheek compartment (medial and lateral components).[10] The superficial middle and lateral cheek compartments can be filled in for final contour improvement.[9,11] The eyebrow is also important in Asian patients. Eyebrow augmentation provides more facial projection and a better setting for the nasofrontal angle. It can also compensate for eyeball protrusion, which is common in Asian faces. When the periorbital area is augmented, the eyeball seems to be set deeper within the face, and the highlights and shadows around the eye are changed.

After the functional zones are set, the highlights can be positioned. Other injection areas are all considered transition zones. The subcutaneous layer and subgalea layers are good choices for this purpose. Especially in the temporal area, some authors proposed deep layer injection for a better morphology. In the current approach, however, this is not necessary. Conceptualizing this area as transitional zone is a good reason to keep the injection within a safe layer, which also produces good, natural results.

The most important transition area lies between the area premaxillary to the cheek and the temporal area. According to the theory of fat compartments, it is the border between the premaxillary compartment and the cheek compartment. When injecting this area, the cannula should go very shallow, just under the dermis, filling in with carefully placed tiny fat droplets. In the frontal view after the surgery, this transition area becomes the new facial contour line (Video 9).

In this series, the entry point of the cannula was placed at the mucosa in the mouth and nostril, which does not risk infection. In the first author's medical practice, the injection site was prepared with povidone iodine before cannula entry as a routine practice. These 2 injection sites were chosen for the following reasons: easy entry, direct access to the planned layer, easy concealment, and quick healing.

Only a few objective measurements were made in this review. The next work is planned to include 3-dimensional scanning. The relationship between body mass index and the fate of fat grafts is also an interesting topic for the further study.

SUMMARY

The author presents a pan-facial fat injection approach to facial contouring in young Asian patients. It is safe, easy to learn, and also provides satisfying aesthetic results. Based on the theory of facial fat compartments, the injection area is classified into functional and transition zones. It is a goal-oriented classification based on anatomic findings. Stable and satisfactory clinical results can be achieved under the guidance of the facial fat compartment theory.

SUPPLEMENTARY DATA

Supplementary data related to this article can be found online at https://doi.org/10.1016/j.cps.2019.08.014.

REFERENCES

1. Peer LA, Walker JC Jr. The behavior of autogenous human tissue grafts; a comparative study. 1. Plast Reconstr Surg (1946) 1951;7:6–23. contd.
2. Coleman SR. Structural fat grafts: the ideal filler? Clin Plast Surg 2001;28:111–9.
3. Peer LA, Walker JC. The behavior of autogenous human tissue grafts. II. Plast Reconstr Surg (1946) 1951;7:73–84.
4. Carpaneda CA, Ribeiro MT. Percentage of graft viability versus injected volume in adipose auto-transplants. Aesthetic Plast Surg 1994;18:17–9.
5. Shi Y, Yuan Y, Dong Z, et al. The fate of fat grafts in different recipient areas: subcutaneous plane, fat pad, and muscle. Dermatol Surg 2016;42:535–42.
6. Amar RE, Fox DM. The facial autologous muscular injection (FAMI) procedure: an anatomically targeted deep multiplane autologous fat-grafting technique using principles of facial fat injection. Aesthetic Plast Surg 2011;35:502–10.
7. Rohrich RJ, Pessa JE. The fat compartments of the face: anatomy and clinical implications for cosmetic surgery. Plast Reconstr Surg 2007;119:2219–27 [discussion 2228–31].
8. Rohrich RJ, Pessa JE, Ristow B. The youthful cheek and the deep medial fat compartment. Plast Reconstr Surg 2008;121:2107–12.
9. Rohrich RJ, Ghavami A, Constantine FC, et al. Lift-and-fill face lift: integrating the fat compartments. Plast Reconstr Surg 2014;133:756e–67e.
10. Ramanadham SR, Rohrich RJ. Newer understanding of specific anatomic targets in the aging face as applied to injectables: superficial and deep facial fat compartments–an evolving target for site-specific facial augmentation. Plast Reconstr Surg 2015;136:49S–55S.
11. Rohrich RJ, Ghavami A, Lemmon JA, et al. The individualized component face lift: developing a systematic approach to facial rejuvenation. Plast Reconstr Surg 2009;123:1050–63.

Fat Grafting for Treatment of Facial Burns and Burn Scars

Nelson Sarto Piccolo, MD[a],*, Mônica Sarto Piccolo, MD, MSc, PhD[a],
Nelson de Paula Piccolo, MD[a], Paulo de Paula Piccolo, MD[a],
Natalia de Paula Piccolo, MD[b], Ricardo Piccolo Daher, MD, MSc[c],
Roberta Piccolo Lobo, MD[a], Silvia Piccolo Daher, MD[b],
Maria Thereza Sarto Piccolo, MD, PhD[d]

KEYWORDS

- Fat grafting • Facial burns • Facial burn sequelae • Wound healing • Scar remodeling

KEY POINTS

- The use of fat grafting has been incorporated into our everyday routine, changing our practice dramatically.
- In relation to facial burns and their sequelae, these changes are more noticeable in the way we treat the resulting scar is taken care of, when present, because fat grafting has also greatly influenced the way hypertrophic scars are treated as a consequence of burn wounds.
- One of the most pleasant surprises in using fat grafts is the minimal incidence (or none) of hypertrophic scarring on the healing of wounds treated with 1 or more sessions of fat grafting.
- In cases whereby no fat grafting was used to treat the acute wound, fat grafting can be used to treat the sequela, and one can note improvement of the scar appearance as well as in volume, as early as 1 to 2 weeks after fat injection/fat delivery.

INTRODUCTION

Fat grafting has become a common procedure in wounds originated from trauma or other causes. Fat contains adipose-derived stem cells and a great variety of growth factors that may have a direct effect in wound healing. Fat grafting has also been used successfully for the management of scars and posttrauma healing fibrosis, scarring, and pain. Adipose-derived stem cells may differentiate into fibroblasts, keratinocytes, and other cells; they may also secrete mediators with neoangiogenic and anti-inflammatory properties. This fact would allow for them to act in all phases of the wound-healing process as it is understood today. Fat on the lipoaspirate can be isolated and/or treated by physical or chemical methods, in the operating room (OR) or in a laboratory setup.[1-8]

As it was used more than a century ago to treat facial deformities, fat grafting, originally (re)introduced in the cephalic segment aiming for improvement in aesthetic aspects of the face and periorbit by Coleman in the early 1990s, soon became one of the main options for disease, trauma, or postsurgery-related deformities.[9,10]

Disclosure: The authors have nothing to disclose.
[a] Division of Plastic Surgery, Pronto Socorro para Queimaduras, Rua 5, n. 439, Setor Oeste, Goiânia, Goiás 74115 060, Brazil; [b] Division of Anesthesiology, Pronto Socorro para Queimaduras, Rua 5, n. 439, Setor Oeste, Goiânia, Goiás 74115 060, Brazil; [c] Division of Outpatient Care, Pronto Socorro para Queimaduras, Rua 5, n. 439, Setor Oeste, Goiânia, Goiás 74115 060, Brazil; [d] Pronto Socorro para Queimaduras, Rua 5, n. 439, Setor Oeste, Goiânia, Goiás 74115 060, Brazil
* Corresponding author.
E-mail address: nelsonpiccolo@grupopiccolo.com.br

plasticsurgery.theclinics.com

PREOPERATIVE EVALUATION AND SPECIAL CONSIDERATIONS

Patients with wounds or scars who are candidates for a fat-grafting procedure at the authors' service are those with the following:

1. Hypertrophic scars that are not improving or not being controlled by pressure garments at 6 or more weeks after healing
2. Burn wounds with 3 weeks or more with no apparent progression to healing
3. Subacute burn wounds or other wounds that are transferred to the authors more than 6 weeks after the accident or wound
4. Venous or diabetic ulcers
5. Decubitus ulcers
6. Wound cavities of any origin (avulsion, drained hematomas, tumor resection, and so forth)
7. Shoulder, wrist, knee, and ankle tendinitis; postfracture "bone pain"; major joint arthrosis

Patients with subacute burn wounds (more than 3 weeks [in the authors' service]) without apparent progression to healing and patients with hypertrophic scarring after healing of a burn or other type of trauma or keloids of any origin are also selected for treatment with fat injection/delivery. Repeat injections (up to 4 injections total) are performed at 7- to 10-day intervals for wounds or at 6- to 8-week intervals for scars.

The use of fat grafting as an adjuvant treatment in acute and subacute burn wounds aims at taking advantage of fat's benefits: a variety of metabolic and regenerative properties, increasing vascularization, and enhancing the tissue regeneration process. When these wounds are treated with (repeated) fat grafting, healing (with minimal fibrosis) is the planned outcome. When treating burn scars, the objective is to decrease the amount of hypertrophy (fibrosis), diminishing the scar thickness, and increasing scar malleability.[11–17]

The actual surgical procedure is performed in the OR, following all rigors and care for sterile procedures.

SURGICAL PROCEDURE
Donor Site Selection

Donor areas are "rotated" as needed, and fat most frequently is obtained from the thighs or lateral upper buttocks, and less frequently, from the abdomen (in the authors' practice, to obtain fat from the abdomen, they first order an ultrasound of the abdominal area to verify the presence [or absence] of wall defects or hernias, which would preclude the use of this area as a donor area).

When necessary, shaving of the pubic area or proximal thigh is performed in the OR, immediately before the procedure. Puncture incisions for the introduction of the liposuction cannula are placed on the midline, at the suprapubic crease, or medial to the femoral pulse, at the inguinal crease, or in the middle axillary line, at the upper border of the iliac bone.

Fat Graft Harvest

The actual volume of harvested lipoaspirate should be at least twice the anticipated volume planned to be injected, and at least 4 times this volume, if one is also planning to have fat delivered over the wound or the scar.

Fat Graft Process

In wounds, the authors use the Coleman technique, repeating injections (and reharvesting) every 7 to 10 days, until healing or until a definite procedure (such as wound closure, skin grafting, flap, or other) is performed. After healing, injections under the scar and fat delivery over the scar are performed at 6- to 8-week intervals, also via the Coleman technique.[18–21]

This approach is also used with patients with scars who seek the authors' service for consultation after being treated elsewhere.

Fat Graft Injection

Patient positioning
Patients are positioned supine when using the abdomen or thighs as donor areas or on lateral decubitus when obtaining fat from the lateral upper thighs. Fat is usually injected and delivered while the patient is supine.

Surgical technique
Fat harvesting and fat injection are sterile surgical procedures and should be performed only in accredited ORs under rigorous, completely sterile technique. Patients are submitted to general anesthesia or regional block.

Recipient site preparation
In patients with scars (healed wounds), the donor area and recipient area are individually prepared and draped in the usual manner.

In patients with open, nonhealed wounds, the donor area is initially prepared and draped, and fat is obtained by liposuction; only then, after the planned amount of fat is obtained, the recipient area is prepared and draped, while the obtained fat is being centrifuged and distributed into various syringes.

Fat is harvested from the patient himself or herself, using a 10-cc Luer Lok syringe, attached to 3-mm canula, with multiple (8–12) distal side openings, with 10-, 15-, or 20-cm length, according to the harvesting site. In children weighing less than 25 kg as well as in women with relatively thin thighs, the authors prefer 20-cc syringes and 2.5-mm cannulas, also multiperforated distally. These cannulas will enforce a higher negative pressure and assure a more even and efficient fat harvesting, respectively. Occasionally, in very small patients (the authors' smallest patient weighted 9.170 kg [an electrical injury to the hand]), it may be necessary to harvest fat from more than 1 donor site.

As recommended by Coleman, 1 or more distally plugged 10-cc syringes containing the obtained fat is centrifuged at 3000 rpm for 3 minutes on a 45° angle centrifuge (1200g). The obtained compound has a top layer of oil, a middle layer of fat (with the Stromal Vascular Fraction within at its lower portion), and an aqueous inferior layer. The top layer of oil is discarded while the plug still is on the syringe. The plug is then removed, and the aqueous layer drains out by gravity. The remaining compound is sequentially injected in an anterograde manner into "insulin" syringes without the plunger, which is then replaced (**Fig. 1**).

Fat Grafting

Using a 16-gauge needle, a perforation is made at an acute angle in healthy skin in the periphery of the wound or the scar. A 1.2-mm outside diameter 70-mm-long cannula already connected to a Luer Lok 1-cc syringe is inserted through the needle puncture hole and (forcefully, if needed) driven immediately under the wound bed or the scar. Fat is then deposited in a retrograde manner, in several "passes" until the entire area is grafted (via as many puncture sites as needed around the periphery of the scar or wound). On average, 1.8 to 2.5 cc of fat are injected per each 10-cm^2 area, and it is necessary to make 25 to 30 "passes" to inject 1 cc.

After the wound area has been completely (under)grafted, the surface of the wound is thoroughly debrided, and fat is deposited in quantity to cover the entire wound. If bone (with or without periosteum), tendons, or nerves are already exposed or exposed after debridement, fat is delivered directly over any or all of these structures. The authors usually debride the wound only after the undersurface has been grafted because in doing so, they avoid having to do multiple punctures around a bleeding wound or running the risk of moving debris along with the injection cannula under the wound.

Similarly, in scar areas, fat also treated by the Coleman technique is injected immediately under the scar. After fat grafting is complete, the scar surface area is treated with a derma roller (usually with 0.5–1.5-mm needle length), or the scar surface may be treated with a fractional CO$_2$ laser, opening "pores" or holes, through the epidermis, into the substance of the scar. Centrifuged fat is then delivered directly to the treated surface (on average, 2.2–3 cc/10 cm^2; **Figs. 2** and **3**).

Very frequently, partial scar removal and fat grafting/fat delivery will be associated. In these cases, the authors perform the partial scar resection first, keeping the resection within the scar substance (trying not to go into subcutaneous tissue). A running nylon suture closes the surgical wound.

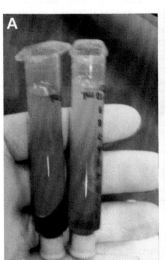
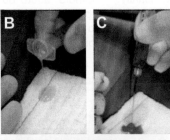
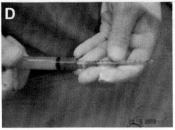

Fig. 1. (*A–D*) Centrifuged lipoaspirate, discarding oil and aqueous layers and filling "insulin" syringe.

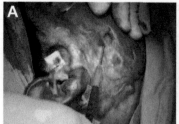
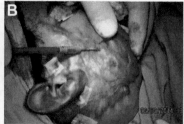
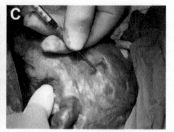

Fig. 2. (*A–C*) Centrifuged fat is injected immediately under the scar, through enough puncture sites entrances, "covering" the entire undersurface of the scar.

Surprisingly, these patients, originally healed from a facial burn with variable amounts of hypertrophic scarring, will NOT hypertrophy at the suture line within the hypertrophic scar. This fact is attributed to the local effect of the fat grafting and the delivered fat previously treated by the Coleman technique (**Fig. 4**).

POSTPROCEDURAL CARE

In wounds, and in scars with fat delivery, a closed dressing is applied with a first layer of petrolatum gauze, followed by several layers of fine-mesh gauze, which is soaked with double-strength Dakin solution (Henry Drysdale Dakin, 1880–1952, English chemist). A bandage finishes the dressing.

Dressings are changed every 2 days. If the delivered fat is firm and adherent on the first dressing, it may stay up to the second dressing change (at 4 days), when it is cleansed with a sponge soaked in normal saline. In scars without fat delivery, a piece of paper tape is placed on each puncture site; it is usually removed in 2 days (**Fig. 5**).

In wounds, it is expected that the delivered fat will turn into another form of live tissue, usually differentiating progressively into granulation tissue, which may or not contract into a healed lesion. When healthy granulation tissue is present,

the area may be partial-thickness skin grafted. If there is still necrotic tissue or exposed noble structures after 7 to 10 days, fat grafting/fat delivery is repeated.

In scars, the delivered fat is cleansed either on the first (if loose) or on the second dressing change (if it was firm and adherent on the first dressing change), also with 2-day intervals.

EXPECTED OUTCOME AND MANAGEMENT OF COMPLICATIONS

All 27 patients with acute or subacute wounds owing to burns or trauma to the face who were submitted to fat grafting/fat delivery healed. Eight patients had frontal bone (5) or malar bone (3) exposure, and all developed a healthy granulation tissue bed after 2 (4 patients) or 3 (4 patients) fat-grafting/fat-delivery procedures. They were then partial-thickness skin grafted, harvesting the skin from the scalp. As the authors have been noticing in the past 8 years in the hundreds of patients treated by them with this technique, minimal or no hypertrophy on healing is the rule.

Although the face is very frequently injured in the authors' acute burn patients (in their institution, about 1 in 8 acute burn patients will have an injury to the face), fat grafting is only occasionally performed in the acute facial burn care. Most of these

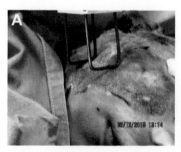
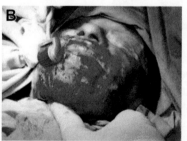
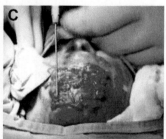

Fig. 3. (*A–C*) After fat grafting, the surface of the scar is treated with a CO_2 laser or a derma roller (0.5–1.5-mm needles), and centrifuged fat is delivered directly over it, using an insulin syringe or a larger-volume syringe, but with the same cannula as for the fat grafting, to ensure an even distribution. Petrolatum gauze and bandages finish the dressing.

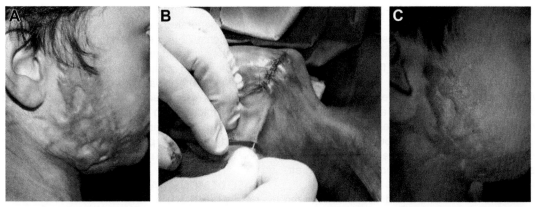

Fig. 4. (*A*) A 4-year-old patient 10 months after ethanol flame burn to the face. (*B*) Partial resection and fat grafting to the undersurface of the resection suture line and the entire scar. (*C*) Result at 2 months. Note the absence of hypertrophy at the suture line.

burns are caused by hot liquids or sudden flame (ethanol or butane); these latter burns usually lead to a more aggressive procedure, generally excision and skin grafting, always using the scalp as donor area.

Fat grafting on the acute burn to the face, at the authors' institution, is more frequently performed when the patient has another burnt area that warrants fat grafting, when several areas are then treated this way, or when a noble structure (nerve, vessel, or bone) is exposed (**Fig. 6**).

Because fat acquisition from very small patients is still infrequent, the authors recommend extreme care in harvesting it, while endeavoring to be symmetric and to obtain deeper fat (under Scarpa fascia) to avoid the occurrence of future superficial irregularities. Also, using slightly higher negative pressure (20-cc syringe) and thinner (2.5 mm) multi- (micro) perforated cannulas will ensure faster and more precise fat harvesting. Assurance of long-term follow-up visits must be provided as the small patient grows.

Complications in fat grafting may be related to the procedure or technique itself, mostly because of physical trauma to underlying structures by the cannula (or other injection device). The authors favor the use of blunt cannulas with distal side openings, connected to a small-volume (1-cc)

syringe, and that fat be injected in a retrograde manner, in multiple passes, depositing multiple, evenly distributed, streaks of fat with less than 2-mm diameter.

In the rare case that a subdermal or suprafascial (deeper) vessel may be injured, local pressure and abortion of the injection on that site should be the immediate action. Ensuing ecchymosis will disappear with time, and the patient must be reassured about the evolution of this most unusual complication.

In scar cases, postoperative edema is a frequent event in the immediate days after the procedure, and the patient must be warned about it.

During their treatment, patients are followed by the entire dedicated team. Support from all related paramedical specialties is constantly provided. In most of the burn sequelae cases, fat grafting is used as a measure to bring relief in scar hypertrophy and restriction. It has proved to be very efficient, occasionally avoiding and frequently postponing scar-removal reconstructive procedures.

All 84 patients with facial scars treated by this technique conveyed improvement after the first fat-grafting procedure: 26 (31%) had a second procedure and 8 (10%) had a third procedure, with noticeable, cumulative improvement

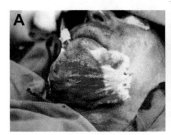
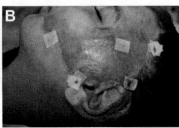

Fig. 5. (*A*) Petrolatum gauze is applied directly over the delivered fat. Fine-mesh gauze and bandages complete the dressing. (*B*) When fat delivery is not performed, paper tape strips are placed at the puncture sites.

after the subsequent fat-grafting/fat-delivery procedures.

One of the main advantages of fat grafting to a scar is the almost immediate perception of decreased hypertrophy and fibrosis. These improvements can also be noticed in scars where centrifuged fat is injected for volume or for recovery of contour appearance, which stays with minimal absorption as well as decreases hypertrophic scarring after wound healing, even when the hypertrophy was already less prominent as in cases that were treated acutely with fat grafting/fat delivery.

This and other related and widely recognized facts are of particular benefit for patients with cicatricial retractions around the eye, nose, and mouth, and in the neck, when reconstructive surgery has frequently failed, with a very large incidence of recurrence.[5,22–26]

REVISIONS OR SUBSEQUENT PROCEDURES

The widely recognized benefits of microneedling have been long recognized by the medical community, mostly for vaccines and drug delivery. The authors coined the term fat delivery based on the successful use of microneedling for other purposes. They postulate that, similarly, microneedling or laser treatment of the scar surface will open pores in enough quantity through the scar surface (epithelium), allowing for delivery of fat and of growth factors contained in fat to penetrate and act directly within the substance of the scar. This fact has certainly brought an additional benefit to the already recognized benefits of subcicatricial injection of fat.[27–34]

The authors have added this technique to every fat grafting to scars, calling it fat delivery. It is performed after fat grafting is done immediately under the scar, when fat also prepared by the Coleman technique is directly delivered to the area, right after microneedling or laser treatment.

It has been reported that micropores in in vivo rat skin generated by microneedles were opened until at least 72 hours after microneedle treatment when they are held under occlusive conditions, for example, using occlusive dressings.

Patients with facial burn scars very frequently will prefer microneedling for fat delivery instead of laser microporing because the laser treatment will yield a temporary wound that is usually not desired by these patients, and microneedling does not usually cause visible wounds (**Fig. 7**).

CASE DEMONSTRATIONS
Case 1

See **Fig. 8**.

Case 2

See **Fig. 9**.

Case 3

See **Fig. 10**.

Case 4

See **Fig. 11**.

DISCUSSION

Fat can easily be grafted in most areas of the face. According to the objective and experience of the surgeon, it will be deposited directly over bone, within the fat compartments, or immediately under the skin. As the authors have demonstrated, it can also be generously applied over microneedled or laser-treated skin, delivering fat directly within the substance of the skin or the scar.[35–38]

Fat injection aimed at improving scars most likely brings improvements through mesenchymal cells and numerous growth factors contained in the lipoaspirate, which contribute to the skin and scar remodeling. In patients with scars that were

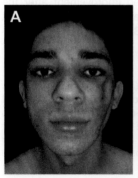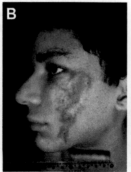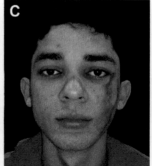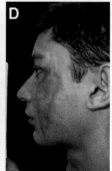

Fig. 6. The same patient in **Fig. 11** 8 weeks after healing and 8 weeks after second fat grafting/fat delivery via microneedling to the scar.

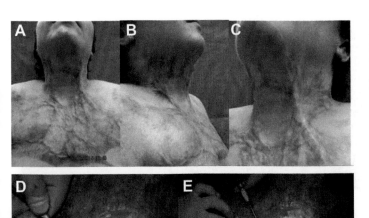

Fig. 7. (*top row*) A 33-year-old patient. (*center row*) Centrifuged fat being delivered after microneedling to the scars and then covered with petrolatum gauze and fine-mesh gauze. (*bottom row*) Appearance 6 months after fat grafting/fat delivery.

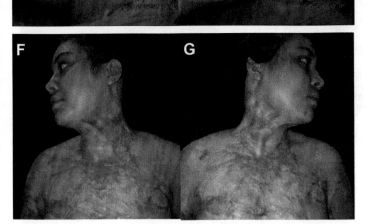

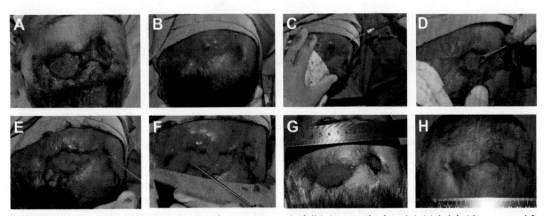

Fig. 8. (*A*) A 45-year-old patient 2 months after a motorcycle fall injury to the head, initial debridement and fat grafting. (*B*) Sixteen days after first procedure. (*C*) Repeat fat grafting under the periphery of the wound. (*D*) Debridement of the wound bed, exposing bone. (*E, F*) Centrifuged fat is delivered to the bony surface of the wound and covered with a petrolatum gauze dressing. (*G*) (*lower right center*) Appearance 22 days after second fat-grafting procedure. (*H*) Healed 30 days after second fat-grafting procedure, appearance 4 weeks after healing.

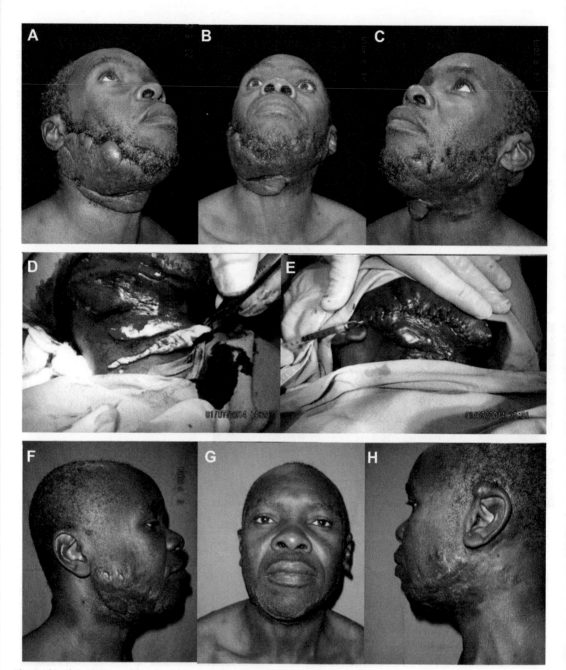

Fig. 9. (*A–C*) A 38-year-old patient 4 years after facial injury with keloid-like scars in a "beard" distribution. (*D, E*) Intralesional resection and fat grafting under the suture line and the entire scar. (*F–H*) Result after 5 similar procedures in 2 years. Note that the resection site suture lines are no longer visible.

treated by this technique, one of the main related improvements was the increase in elasticity and malleability of the scar tissue as well as for its significant decrease in volume and thickness. This fact could be partially due to the marked increase in the number of elastic fibers, easily perceived microscopically in postinjection scar samples, in consequence of these injections.

This improvement could be related to the number of injections and/or the time elapsed after injection, because there are definite, progressive, and cumulative changes after repeat injections.

There are many publications in the literature where investigators indicate that the method of harvesting and the way that the lipoaspirate is handled, or enriched, or injected could influence

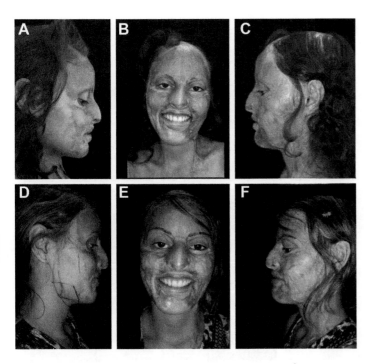

Fig. 10. (*A–C*) A 16-year-old patient who suffered a flame burn to the face and body at age 2 (previously treated elsewhere). (*D–F*) Results at 4 months after 2 fat-grafting procedures performed at 4-month intervals. Note improvement in left lateral canthus in the orbital area, at both nostril-nasolabial fold junction and left oral commissure.

the result of each specific fat-injection procedure. The authors believe that the Coleman technique provides a rather standardized method, with a very short learning curve for the surgeon and with an easy-to-learn routine by the entire surgical team. Procedures practiced and results presented by different surgeons will make these results easier to compare, when the harvesting and preparation of the fat are done with a similar technique or method, such as the widely known Coleman technique.

Because the technique of blunt cannula insertion optimizes the release of scar retraction, this may also play a part in the analgesic effect of this treatment method. This finding is related in published evidence that supports current theories of mesenchymal stem cell's regenerative and anti-inflammatory properties responsible for scar healing.

The logical sequential procedure for fat grafting/fat delivery to scars is the scar-removal procedure. The authors favor the use of tissue expansion, which very frequently is a sequence of several partial scar removals, which follow each tissue expansion. It is also very important to warn the patients that they will have access to these operations, and the authors' multidisciplinary team considers the entire sequence when caring for a patient, regardless of whether the patient was originally treated in the acute phase at their institution.

One must always consider the patient's desire as the main direction for reconstructive surgery indication and recommendation. As scars are removed, the patients tend to forget how large or how deforming the actual scar was, and then migrate to wishing changes aiming at more aesthetic concepts, like apparently minor changes

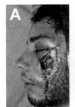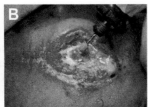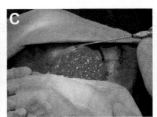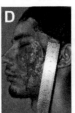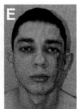

Fig. 11. (*A*) A 21-year-old patient 26 days after motorcycle accident and severe burn to the face, with exposure of malar bone. (*B–D*) Debridement (soft tissue and bone) and fat grafting/fat delivery to the wound. (*E*) Appearance at healing, after 3 fat-grafting procedures, 2 bone debridements, and scalp partial thickness skin grafting.

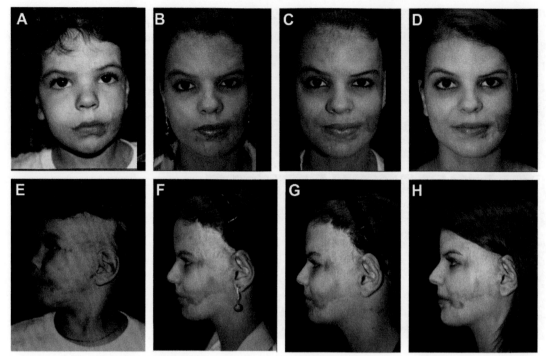

Fig. 12. (*A, E*) Patient suffered flame burn at age 2.5. (*B, F*) Appearance after tissue expansion of scalp and neck/mandibular skin with partial facial scar removal. (*C, G*) Result after first fat grafting. (*D, H*) Appearance after second fat-grafting/fat-delivery procedure. Note significant improvement in position and appearance of the left corner of the mouth and left eyebrow as well as scar surface and texture. Patient did not desire further reconstruction.

within areas of larger scars. They may also desire immediate "minor" improvements as major surgery is programmed, which could be obtained by 1 or more fat-grafting/fat-delivery procedures.

It may also occur that the patient may wish exactly the opposite, when the patient would like to have a "larger" operation (like a tissue expansion with 2 or more expanders in the same cavity), which would yield a more visible and ample result than a relatively "minor" procedure such as fat grafting; this desire usually occurs when treating scars that usually do not compromise major orifices (such as mouth, nose, or eye) and are "just" surface scars in the face (or other areas of the body). In these cases, the authors may perform both procedures, at the same time, or as tissue expansion is happening, adding benefit to the final result. Older children and adults will frequently desire changes in procedures as they notice the improvement (**Fig. 12**).

SUMMARY

Fat grafting as an adjuvant treatment of burn and other wounds in the face favors healing, while decreasing the usual healing time, as well as fostering lesser to practically no hypertrophic

scarring. When used under scars and/or immediately over them, it diminishes fibrosis, diminishing scar thickness, and allowing for more pliability of the skin and for recovering of the normal mimic and contour. For these benefits to occur, there may be a need for repeat fat injections at certain intervals, until the desired result is obtained or other type of reconstructive procedure is performed.

ACKNOWLEDGEMENTS

The authors would like to thank the most important assistance of Dr. Altamiro Vieira, MD in the photographic documentation of these cases.

REFERENCES

1. Zuk PA, Zhu M, Mizuno H, et al. Multilineage cells from human adipose tissue: implications for cell-based therapies. Tissue Eng 2001;7:211.
2. Zuk PA, Zhu M, Ashjian P, et al. Human adipose tissue is a source of multipotent stem cells. Mol Biol Cell 2002;13:4279–95.
3. Fujimura J, Ogawa R, Mizuno H, et al. Neural differentiation of adipose-derived stem cells isolated from

GFP transgenic mice. Biochem Biophys Res Commun 2005;333(1):116–21.

4. Dominici M, Le Blanc K, Mueller I, et al. Minimal criteria for defining multipotent mesenchymal stromal cells, the International Society for Cellular Therapy position statement. Cryotherapy 2006;8:315–7.

5. Rigotti G, Marchi A, Galiè M, et al. Clinical treatment of radiotherapy tissue damage by lipoaspirate transplant: a healing process mediated by adipose derived adult stem cells. Plast Reconstr Surg 2007;119:1409–22.

6. Gimble JM, Katz AJ, Foster SJ. Adipose-derived stem cells for regenerative medicine. Circ Res 2007;100:1249–60.

7. Akita S, Akino K, Hirano A, et al. Non-cultured autologous adipose-derived stem cells therapy for chronic radiation injury. Stem Cells Int 2010 [Article ID: 532704].

8. Brown SA, Levi B, Lequeux C, et al. Basic science review on adipose tissue for clinicians. Plast Reconstr Surg 2010;126:1936–46.

9. Benmoussa N, Hansen K, Charlier P. Use of fat grafts in facial reconstruction on the wounded soldiers from the first World War (WWI) by Hippolyte Morestin (1869-1919). Ann Plast Surg 2017;79:420–2.

10. Baum SH, Rieger G, Pförtner R, et al. Correction of whistle deformity using autologous free fat grafting: first results of a pilot study and review of the literature. Oral Maxillofac Surg 2017;21:409–18.

11. Yoshimura K, Sato K, Aoi N, et al. Cell-assisted lipotransfer for facial lipoatrophy: efficacy of clinical use of adipose-derived stem cells. Dermatol Surg 2008;34:1178–85.

12. Viard R, Bouguilla J, Voulhaume D, et al. La lipostructure dans les sequelles de brulures facials. Ann Chir Plast Esthet 2012;57:217–29.

13. Sultan SM, Barr JS, Butala P, et al. Fat grafting accelerates revascularization and decreases fibrosis following thermal injury. J Plast Reconstr Aesthet Surg 2012;65:219–27.

14. Carpaneda CA, Ribeiro MT. Study of histologic alterations and viability of adipose grafts in humans. Aesthetic Plast Surg 1993;17:43–7.

15. Kim W, Park BS, Sung JH, et al. Wound healing effect of adipose-derived stem cells: a critical role of secretory factors on human dermal fibroblasts. J Dermatol Sci 2007;48:15–24.

16. Lolli P, Malleo G, Rigotti G. Treatment of chronic anal fissures and associated stenosis by autologous adipose tissue transplant: a pilot study. Dis Colon Rectum 2010;53:460–6.

17. Bene MD, Pozzi MR, Rovati L, et al. Autologous fat grafting for scleroderma-induced digital ulcers. An effective technique in patients with systemic sclerosis. Handchir Mikrochir Plast Chir 2014;46:242–7.

18. Coleman SR. The technique of periorbital lipoinfiltration. Oper Tech Plast Reconstr Surg 1994;1(3):120–6.

19. Coleman SR. Long-term survival of fat transplants: controlled demonstrations. Aesthetic Plast Surg 1995;19:421–5.

20. Coleman SR. Structural fat grafts: the ideal filler? Clin Plast Surg 2001;28:111–9.

21. Coleman SR, editor. Structural fat grafting. St Louis (MO): Quality Medical Publishing; 2004.

22. Bourne DA, Thomas RD, Bliley J, et al. Amputation-site soft-tissue restoration using adipose stem cell therapy. Plast Reconstr Surg 2018;142:1349–52.

23. Luck J, Smith OJ, Malik D, et al. Protocol for a systematic review of autologous fat grafting for wound healing. Syst Rev 2018;7:99.

24. Bashir MM, Sohail M, Bashir A, et al. Outcome of conventional adipose tissue grafting for contour deformities of face and role of ex vivo expanded adipose tissue-derived stem cells in treatment of such deformities. J Craniofac Surg 2018;29:1143–7.

25. Klinger M, Marazzi M, Vigo D, et al. Fat injection for cases of severe burn outcomes: a new perspective of scar remodeling and reduction. Aesthetic Plast Surg 2008;32:465–9.

26. Pallua N, Baroncini A, Alharbi Z, et al. Improvement of facial scar appearance and microcirculation by autologous lipofilling. J Plast Reconstr Aesthet Surg 2014;67:1033–7.

27. Vandervoort J, Ludwig A. Microneedles for transdermal drug delivery: a minireview. Front Biosci 2008;13:1711–5.

28. Kaushik S, Hord AH, Denson DD, et al. Lack of pain associated with microfabricated microneedles. Anesth Analg 2001;92:502–4.

29. Prausnitz MR. Microneedles for transdermal drug delivery. Adv Drug Deliv Rev 2004;56:581–7.

30. Kalluri H, Banga AK. Formation and closure of microchannels in skin following microporation. Pharm Res 2010;28:82–94.

31. Li K, Yoo KH, Byun HJ, et al. The microneedle roller is an effective device for enhancing transdermal drug delivery. Int J Dermatol 2012;51:1137–9. 52.

32. Kim YC, Park JH, Prausnitz MR. Microneedles for drug and vaccine delivery. Adv Drug Deliv Rev 2012;64:1547–68.

33. Van der Maaden K, Jiskoot W, Bouwstra J. Microneedle technologies for (trans)dermal drug and vaccine delivery. J Control Release 2012;161:645–55.

34. Soltani-Arabshahi R, Wong JW, Duffy KL, et al. Facial allergic granulomatous reaction and systemic hypersensitivity associated with microneedle therapy for skin rejuvenation. JAMA Dermatol 2014;150:68–72.

35. Chen H, Zhang Q, Qiu Q, et al. Autologous fat graft for the treatment of sighted posttraumatic enophthalmos and sunken upper eyelid. Ophthalmic Plast Reconstr Surg 2018;34:381–6.

36. Diepenbrock RM, Green JM 3rd. Autologous fat transfer for maxillofacial reconstruction. Atlas Oral Maxillofac Surg Clin North Am 2018;26:59–68.

37. Foubert P, Zafra D, Liu M, et al. Autologous adipose-derived regenerative cell therapy modulates development of hypertrophic scarring in a red Duroc porcine model. Stem Cell Res Ther 2017;8:261.

38. Marten TJ, Elyassnia D. Fat grafting in facial rejuvenation. Clin Plast Surg 2015;42:219–52.

Fat Grafting for Treatment of Facial Scars

Marco Klinger, MD[a],*, Francesco Klinger, MD[b], Fabio Caviggioli, MD[b], Luca Maione, MD[a], Barbara Catania, MD[a], Alessandra Veronesi, MD[a], Silvia Giannasi, MD[a], Valeria Bandi, MD[a], Micol Giaccone, MD[a], Mattia Siliprandi, MD[a], Federico Barbera, MD[a], Andrea Battistini, MD[a], Andrea Lisa, MD[a], Valeriano Vinci, MD[a]

KEYWORDS

- Lipofilling • Face • Scars • Burns • Autologous fat grafting

KEY POINTS

- Lipofilling has become an important tool for plastic surgeons in treating all the diseases resulting in scars.
- Fat grafting has shown to have a great regenerative potential due to the presence of the mesenchymal stem cells that allow scar remodeling and improve the quality of the scar tissue.
- One of the possible uses of lipofilling is the treatment of facial scars, especially if derived from burns, trauma, degenerative diseases, and radiotherapy.

INTRODUCTION

Autologous fat grafting, also known as fat auto-transplantation or lipofilling, is one of the most interesting and useful techniques in plastic surgery and is now used for both cosmetic and reconstructive surgical procedures. Adipose tissue is a connective tissue full of different cells, including the mesenchymal stem cells, which have a primary role in the regenerative purposes of the autologous fat grafting. Fat stem cells are not the primordial stem cells as the ones stored in the bone marrow, thymus, or spleen. They are more likely pluripotent fibroblasts or mesenchymal cells (third-generation differentiating cells) harvested from around vessels and nerves. Similar to other stem cells, the mesenchymal stem cells possess the 2 main properties of a stem cell: self-renewal and potency (the capacity to differentiate into specialized cell types).

The concept of autologous fat grafting was first described in 1893 by Neuber and subsequently by Hollander (1912), Neuhof (1923), and Josef (1931), to treat complex congenital malformations, traumatic wounds, and postoncological demolishing procedures. One of the leaders in fat transplantation is Sidney Coleman MD, who described a new method to improve the survival of the transplanted mesenchymal stem cells in the early 1990s.[1–7] Rigotti and colleagues[8] in 1997 first used fat injection for the treatment of radiodermatitis.

PREOPERATIVE EVALUATION AND SPECIAL CONSIDERATIONS

Before performing a lipofilling procedure, all patients need a clinical assessment and routine preoperative examination; it is important to gauge the mindset and goals of the patient and inform that

Disclosure Statement: The authors have nothing to disclose.
[a] Plastic Surgery Unit, Department of Medical Biotechnology and Translational Medicine BIOMETRA, Humanitas Clinical and Research Hospital, Reconstructive and Aesthetic Plastic Surgery School, University of Milan, Via Manzoni 56, Rozzano, Milan 20090, Italy; [b] Plastic Surgery Unit, MultiMedica Holding S.p.A., Reconstructive and Aesthetic Plastic Surgery School, University of Milan, Via Milanese, 300, Sesto San Giovanni, Milan 20099, Italy
* Corresponding author.
E-mail address: marco.klinger@humanitas.it

Clin Plastic Surg 47 (2020) 131–138
https://doi.org/10.1016/j.cps.2019.09.002

the volume of the fat may fluctuate with weight loss or gain. In case of scar treatment, preoperative markings of the face are mandatory, asking the patient to note the areas of greater tension and impairment to daily life activities and joint movements.[9]

There are multiple graft donor sites and, up to now, there are no data that support one site is better than others. After the fat is harvested and processed, it can be grafted in the face. There are multiple different areas of the face that can be treated with autologous fat grafting, such as the glabella, forehead, temporal fossa hollows, labiomental crease, lips, prejowl sulci, and even earlobes. In these areas the presence of a scar can create different grades of volume deficit that can be successfully treated with lipofilling. It is known that areas of the face that have least motion and thicker overlying tissues have the best survival of the transferred fat (cheek, nasolabial folds, and malar region). On the other side, areas under motion and thinner preexisting fat content (such as the perioral region, the lips, and the marionettes) can have variable results after lipofilling.

Nowadays fat grafting is becoming mandatory in several procedures. The reason why it has become so popular is because it is a simple, safe, and repeatable procedure that can be used to treat virtually every part of the body, including the face, for multiple clinical applications:

- Scar release
- Restoring of improving skin quality
- Improvement of radiodystrophic skin
- Volume and contour
- Treatment of pain syndromes
- Treatment of degenerative diseases
- Wound healing
- Aesthetic purposes

SURGICAL TECHNIQUE

The authors' technique, similar to the one described by Coleman, is based on the following steps: under local anesthesia and sedation, the donor areas (including the thighs, flanks, or abdomen) are incised with a 15-blade scalpel and infiltrated with a blunt cannula filled with anesthetic solution (the authors' group uses 100 mL saline solution, 10 mL of levobupivacaine 7.5 mg/mL, 20 mL of mepivacaine 10 mg/mL, and 0.5 mL epinephrine 1 mg/mL). Adipose tissue is then harvested using the same skin incisions with blunt cannulas of 2 to 3 mm in diameter of variable length (between 15 and 23 cm). The cannula is connected with a Luer-lock syringe. After creating a negative pressure, the cannula is advanced and retracted with radial movements inside the whole donor area. The harvested tissue is then centrifuged at 3000 rpm for 3 minutes.

This step is extremely important because it allows the separation of the unwanted components (oil, blood, local anesthetic, and other noncellular material) from the pure fat. Centrifugation increases the content of adipose-derived stem cells, reduces the amount of proinflammatory blood cells, and concentrates a higher number of viable cells with regenerative potential. The authors recently demonstrated that centrifugation does not impair cell viability[10] and is able to concentrate a higher number of cells (**Figs. 1** and **2**). The purified fat is transferred into a 1-mL syringe Luer-lock that allows a good control of the amount of fat injected and better handling.

The fat can be injected using needles or blunt cannulas. In the authors' experience blunt cannulas are not perfect instruments; their group believes that the best choice is an 18-gauge angiographic sharp needle (Cordis Corp., Bridgewater, NJ, USA) and the Seldinger technique.[11] Using a sharp needle allows the interruption of scar tissue, obtaining a "new space" where the fat can be grafted. This technique seems to allow better fat graft survival, increase graft uptake, and minimize the possibility of oil-forming cysts. Placement of the fat in small aliquots is the key of the Coleman technique because it ensures the proximity of the injected fat to a blood supply and allows the fat to anchor to the recipient tissue. These aliquots should be placed as the cannula is withdrawn, and no more than 0.1 mL of fat should be placed with each pass. In fact, if fat is injected in a bolus, fat cells will be clumped together and only those on the periphery of the injected area will have

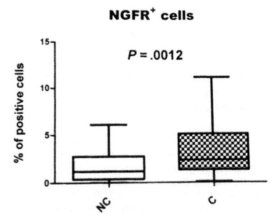

Fig. 1. Number of recovered cells in the noncentrifuged fraction (NCF) and the centrifuged fraction (CF) samples. The CF samples contained a significantly greater number of cells.

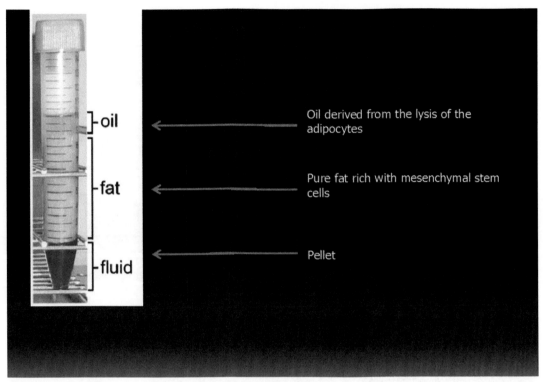

oil — Oil derived from the lysis of the adipocytes

fat — Pure fat rich with mesenchymal stem cells

fluid — Pellet

Fig. 2. The 3 layers after centrifugation.

contact with the recipient tissue and will be more likely to survive (**Fig. 3**).

POSTOPERATIVE CARE

The treated areas are covered with paper patches for 5 days and the patient is asked to avoid pressure and friction to limit the displacement of fat. The skin incisions in the donor areas are sutured with 4/0 Vicryl. Abdomen and trochanteric areas are usually medicated with an elastic-compressive dressing and kept in place for 5 days to prevent any risk of hematoma.

EXPECTED OUTCOME AND MANAGEMENT OF COMPLICATIONS

The complications of this technique are limited and rare. The most common are infections (cellulitis), prolonged swelling, intravascular injections, fat necrosis, ecchymosis, contour irregularities/asymmetries, and overgrafting. In case of excessive fat grafting, the only possible treatment is a microliposuction of the area involved.[12]

The volume retention after grafting is unpredictable and the percentages are very different in the scientific literature. For this reason, an overcorrection of 20% to 30% should be recommended due to the expected resorption rate. The use of

additives such as stromal vascular fraction and growth factors such as platelet-rich plasma may increase the predictability of fat grafting, but there are still many doubts about this. Recent studies have shown that fat grafting to the face enriched by stromal vascular fraction (SVF) can lead to a better retention, with a survival of the graft around 68%. In addition, there is evidence that the fat volume retention is improved with increase in number of cells in the SVF.[13]

REVISION OR SUBSEQUENT PROCEDURES

Lipofilling has proved to be a safe procedure that can be repeated several times, especially in case of unsatisfactory aesthetic or functional outcomes after the first treatment. Studies have shown that fat grafting enhances the vascularity of the involved area; for this reason, every time fat is grafted, the percentage of cells that are able to survive tends to increase. Besides, it has been seen that weight gain can cause an enlargement of the fat graft, which can lead to poor aesthetic results, especially on the face. In these situations, as in all the situations of overgrafting, a microliposuction is required in order to rebalance the excessive fat injected. Finally, in specific situations, fat grafting can be performed in association with other surgical procedures (Z-plasty, surgical scar

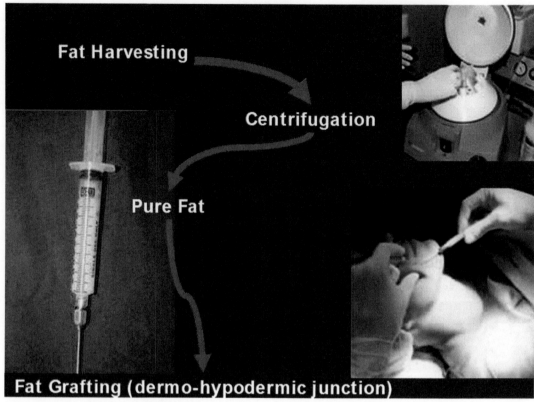

Fig. 3. Different steps of lipofilling.

release, scar revision) with the intent of improving the quality of the scar.

CASE DEMONSTRATIONS

Case 1. See **Fig. 4**.
Case 2. See **Fig. 5**.
Case 3. See **Fig. 6**.

DISCUSSION

The most common surgical procedures for treating the scars are traditional Z-plasty, dermoepidermal grafts, and V-Y flaps, whereas the most common medical and conservative therapies are elastic-compressive garments, topical silicone sheets, physiotherapy, splint, corticosteroid injection in scar area, laser therapy, cryotherapy, and radiotherapy. These procedures, especially the surgical ones, may often lead to satisfactory results but frequently show a high tendency to relapse. Autologous fat grafting has shown to be an excellent solution in terms of good results and reduced risk of relapse.

Autologous fat grafting can be used in every area of the face to improve mature scars and

fibrotic tissues in terms of skin texture, color, volume, softness, and quality of skin patterns. The versatility of this procedure makes it useful not only as a filler but also as a rejuvenating-regenerative technique. The biological effect of the autologous fat graft is due to the presence of mesenchymal multipotent stem cells that are responsible for remodeling through engraftment and differentiation. This effect leads to molecular changes in the microenvironment of the scars (**Fig. 7**). At the basis of the scar remodeling process there is the local action of cytokines, growth factors, angiogenic factors, enzymes, and cellular component stored in the lipoaspirate leading to neoangiogenesis in the fibrotic tissue.[14] From a histologic point of view, autologous fat graft has shown the ability to regenerate the dermis and subcutaneous tissue. Furthermore, it also has the ability to improve the quality of the dermal and dermo-hypodermic areas of the scars, by increasing the amount of the fat layer that poorly regenerates during tissue repair after any type of trauma.

Lipofilling has shown to be an excellent solution to treat retractile and painful scars of the face, especially the ones compromising the regular daily

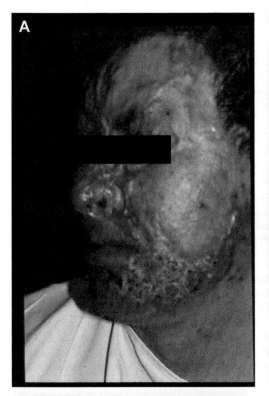

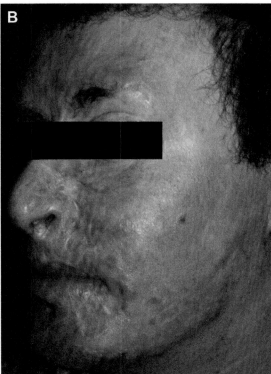

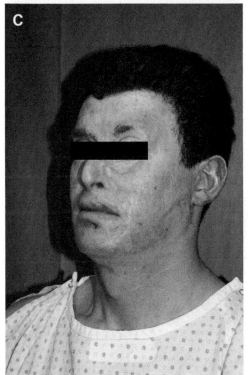

Fig. 4. Patient with a burn scar of the face treated with multiple lipofilling procedures. The skin quality, the texture, the color, and the pliability have improved throughout the time. (*A*) It is possible to see the burn outcomes before fat grafting (view of the patient 8 years after burn injuries;note the left alar nose retraction and right upper lip tension). (*B*) The same patient after 2 lipofillings. (*C*) The same patient after 3 treatments. Note the further improvement of skin texture and correct repositioning of the alar nose and right upper lip.

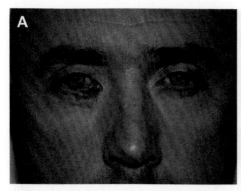
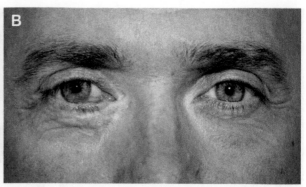

Fig. 5. Patient with medial cicatricial ectropion of the right eye treated with lipofilling. (*A*) The preoperative scenario. (*B*) The same patient 1 year after treatment with fat injection. Note the complete functional recovery with excellent cosmetic results. (*From* Caviggioli F, Klinger F, Villani F, et al. Correction of cicatricial ectropion by autologous fat graft. Aesthetic Plast Surg. 2008;32(3):556–7; with permission.)

activities or mobility of the joints. The nature of the scars can be very different: they can arise from burn injuries, trauma, domestic accident, radiotherapy, and surgery procedures.

The authors' group has obtained great results in treating different types of facial scars, as the contracted scars causing microstomia (especially when deriving from burn scars), eversion of the lip, cicatricial ectropion, nasal valve collapse, and mimic deficits. Sometimes these scars can reduce the range of passive and active motion of one or multiple joints. The results of lipofilling can be seen starting from 3 months after the procedure, in terms of better scar color, pliability, thickness, relief, itching, pain, scar vascularization, and pigmentation (see **Fig. 4**).[15] Indeed autologous fat graft makes the skin softer, more flexible, and extensible; besides the color seems similar to the surrounding skin. The release of scar bridles (both the most superficial and the deepest ones) improves the mobility of the body district involved, in particular joints, the eyelids, the nasal valve, and the mouth, and can lead to a partial restoration of facial mimic (kissing, smiling, frowning, and other mood expression). In patients with great skin depression caused by retracting scars, the use of the autologous fat graft often fills these volume deficits, allowing to achieve excellent cosmetic results and also allowing the patient to change the face contour.

The authors' group has also recently used autologous fat grafting to treat a case of cicatricial ectropion. Ectropion is an outward rotation of the lower eyelid and can be divided into 5 broad clinical categories: congenital, involutional, cicatricial, paralytic, and mechanical. The authors focused on the cicatricial ectropion, the most common etiological factor of which is the anterior lamella shortening. The cicatricial ectropion can be corrected

by lipofilling, especially when the standard dermoepidermal graft leads to a poor functional and cosmetic result (see **Fig. 5**).[16,17]

Lipofilling has numerous advantages and few disadvantages in treating the scars of the face.[18–22] The use of the autologous fat grafting helps the skin to become softer, more flexible, and extensible, and the color seems similar to the surrounding unharmed skin. It improves the mobility of the body district treated, in particular joints, eyelids, nasal valve, and mouth; it also increases the possibility for the patient to have a partial restoration of facial mimic (kiss, smile, and other mood expressions). Lipofilling can also restore volume deficits. From a histologic point of view, autologous fat graft has shown the ability to regenerate the dermis and subcutaneous tissue (angiogenesis and new collagen deposition). Unfortunately, the deep mechanism of tissue quality improvement, the rate of fat graft

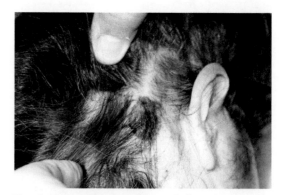

Fig. 6. Preoperative marking of the trigger point where the nerve entrapment is located. This is the area where fat is grafted and can exert its effects by releasing the nervous fibers and reducing the pain related to cervical neuropathic neuralgia.

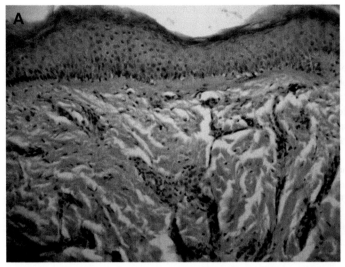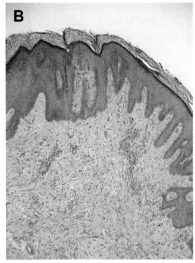

Fig. 7. Reconstruction of an example of ridges and dermal papillae in a posttreatment biopsy (*B*) compared with baseline (*A*) (hematoxylin and eosin staining, original magnification 20x, insert 4x).

resorption, and how the same treatment can give unpredictable results in different patients are still unclear.

One of the most interesting diseases that can be treated with lipofilling is the cervical neuropathic neuralgia when deriving from scars (off-label use). Cervical headache is defined as a pain referred to the occipital nerve sensory territory. There are 2 different types of cervical neuropathic neuralgia accepted in the scientific literature: the chronic cervical headache (CCH) and occipital neuralgia (ON). CCH is characterized by a nonthrobbing pain originating posteriorly in the neck and spreading toward the front-orbital area; it is usually exacerbated by external pressure on specific trigger points. ON is characterized by a paroxysmal shooting or stabbing pain referred in the sensory territory of the great occipital nerves. The pain originates in the suboccipital region and spreads to the vertex. The pathophysiology is still unclear, even though a possible cause could be a myofascial spasm that is present together with a focal entrapment of the occipital nerve due to local fibrosis. The most frequent site of occipital nerve entrapment is located at the level of the passage of occipital nerve at the trapezoid tunnel. During time different nonsurgical and surgical options have been proposed to treat this disease. Nonsurgical ones include physical therapy such as massage or local heat, nonsteroidal antiinflammatory drugs, myorelaxants, and oral anticonvulsant drugs. Surgical decompression of C2 nerve root, ganglion, and/or postganglionic nerve may be considered when the pain is chronic,

severe, and unresponsive to conservative treatments. Recently the use of the autologous fat grafting has been proposed to treat patients with cervical neuropathic neuralgia, because lipofilling has shown to be an excellent choice in scar and fibrosis treatment. The fat needs to be injected in the proximity of the nerve emergence, which is generally 3 cm below the occipital notch and 1.5 cm lateral to the midline (see **Fig. 6**). Eighty percent of the patients undergoing fat grafting for ON or CCH experienced a significant clinical response with a good pain relief and an important improvement in quality of life.[23]

SUMMARY

Autologous fat grafting can be used in almost every area of the face to improve mature scars and fibrotic tissues in terms of skin texture, color, volume, softness, and quality of skin patterns. The versatility of this procedure makes it useful not only as a filler but also as a rejuvenating-regenerative technique. However, the exact mechanism of tissue quality improvement, the rate of fat graft resorption, and how the same treatment can give unpredictable results in different patients are still unclear.

REFERENCES

1. Coleman SR. Facial augmentation with structural fat grafting. Clin Plast Surg 2006;33:567.
2. Neuber F. Fat transplantation. Chir Kongr Verhandl Dsch Gesellch Chir 1893;22:66.

3. Neuhof H. The transplantation of tissues. New York: Appleton et Comp; 1923.

4. Josef J. Nasenplastic und sonstige Gesichtplstik nebst einem anhang ueber mammaplstik und einige weitere Operationem aus dem Gebiete der ausserem K-rperplastik, ein atlas und ein lehrbuch. Berlin; 1931.

5. Billings E Jr, May JW Jr. Historical review and present status of free fat graft autotransplantation in plastic and reconstructive surgery. Plast Reconstr Surg 1989;83:368.

6. Von Heimburg D, Hemmrich K, Haydarlioglu S, et al. Comparison of viable cell yield from excised versus aspired adipose tissue. Cells Tissues Organs 2004; 178:87.

7. Coleman SR. Long-term survival of fat transplants: controlled demonstrations. Aesthetic Plast Surg 1995;19:421.

8. Rigotti G, Marchi A, Galiè M, et al. Clinical treatment of radiotherapy tissue damage by lipoaspirate transplant: a healing process mediated by adipose-derived adult stem cells. Plast Reconstr Surg 2007;119:1409–22.

9. Klinger M, Lisa A, Klinger F, et al. Regenerative approach to scars, ulcers and related problems with fat grafting. Clin Plast Surg 2015;42(3):345–52.

10. Ibatici A, Caviggioli F, Valeriano V, et al. Comparison of cell number, viability,phenotypic profile, clonogenic, and proliferative potential of adipose-derived stem cell populations between centrifuged and noncentrifuged fat. Aesthetic Plast Surg 2014; 38(5):985–93.

11. Maione L, Vinci V, Klinger M, et al. Autologous fat graft by needle: analysis of complications after 1000 patients. Ann Plast Surg 2015;74(3):277–80.

12. Caviggioli F, Forcellini D, Vinci V, et al. Employment of needles: a different technique for fat placement. Plast Reconstr Surg 2012;130(2):373e–4e.

13. Schendel SA. Reply: enriched autologous facial fat grafts in aesthetic surgery: 3d volumetric results. Plast Reconstr Surg 2016;137(3):639e.

14. Carelli S, Colli M, Vinci V, et al. Mechanical activation of adipose tissue and derived mesenchymal stem cells: novel anti-inflammatory properties. Int J Mol Sci 2018;19(1) [pii:E267].

15. Klinger M, Marazzi M, Vigo D, et al. Fat injection for cases of severe burn outcomes: a new perspective of scar remodeling and reduction. Aesthetic Plast Surg 2008;32(3):465–9.

16. Caviggioli F, Klinger F, Villani F, et al. Correction of cicatricial ectropion by autologous fat graft. Aesthetic Plast Surg 2008;32(3):555–7.

17. Lupo F, Ioppolo L, Pino D, et al. Lipograft in cicatricial ectropion. Ann Ital Chir 2016;87:466–9.

18. Klinger M, Caviggioli F, Klinger FM, et al. Autologous fat graft in scar treatment. J Craniofac Surg 2013; 24(5):1610–5.

19. Harp A, Liu YF, Inman JC, et al. Autologous lipoinjection in Parry-Romberg syndrome. Ear Nose Throat J 2018;97(6):151–2.

20. Lee ZH, Khoobehi K, Chiu ES. Autologous fat grafting for treatment of facial atrophy in Behcet's disease: a case report. J Plast Reconstr Aesthet Surg 2013;66(12):1759–62.

21. Gheisari M, Ahmadzadeh A, Nobari N, et al. Autologous fat grafting in the treatment of facial scleroderma. Dermatol Res Pract 2018;2018: 6568016.

22. Guibert M, Franchi G, Ansari E, et al. Fat graft transfer in children's facial malformations: a prospective three-dimensional evaluation. J Plast Reconstr Aesthet Surg 2013;66(6):799–804.

23. Gaetani P, Klinger M, Levi D, et al. Treatment of chronic headache of cervical origin with lipostructure: an observational study. Headache 2013;53(3): 507–13.

Microfat and Lipoconcentrate for the Treatment of Facial Scars

Norbert Pallua, MD, PhD[a],*, Bong-Sung Kim, MD[b]

KEYWORDS

- Lipofilling • Adipose-derived stem cells • Emulsified fat • Scar treatment • Nanofat
- Regenerative medicine

KEY POINTS

- Growth factors and adipose-derived stem cells are the molecular and cellular sources respectively for the regenerative effect of fat grafts.
- The addition of platelet-rich plasma may support the effect of fat grafts.
- Facial scars require accurate preoperative evaluation in order to use the right technique.
- Emulsified nanofat, also called lipoconcentrate, is particularly useful in facial scar treatment due to its low volume and high content of regenerative cells.

INTRODUCTION

The regenerative effect of adipose tissue and its inherent cells is unquestioned, as intense research efforts over many years have shown. The source for the reparative function of adipose tissue is believed to be of cellular as well as molecular nature. The multipotent mesenchymal stem/stromal cells within adipose tissue, called adipose-derived stem cells (ASCs), are widely accepted as cells with broad differentiation and proliferation capacity. Moreover, soluble factors, including enzymes, cytokines, and growth factors, add to the tissue modulation.[1]

Besides cosmetic facial and body contouring, fat grafting has emerged as a credible solution for the reconstructive treatment of facial scars in particular. Facial scars, often perceived as extremely disfiguring as well as stigmatizing for patients and at the same time tedious to treat, seem to greatly benefit from the regenerative properties of autologous fat tissue.

In the present work, the technique for regenerative fat grafting of facial scars as applied and optimized over many years by the first author is presented and discussed in detail.

PREOPERATIVE EVALUATION AND SPECIAL CONSIDERATIONS

A careful patient selection is the first and probably the most important step of successful treatment. Although fat grafting is an undeniably powerful tool in plastic surgery, it cannot eradicate scars completely, as requested by some patients. Thus, thorough consultation, even more so in patients with unrealistic expectations, is mandatory.

Fat grafting should be considered for patients with mature, flat, and even facial scars at the level of the skin. Also, mature scars with signs of moderate or even severe retraction are good indications. Finally, mature scars with loss or disturbed pigmentation are regarded as feasible

Disclosure Statement: Both authors declare no conflict of interest. B.-S. Kim was supported by the Deutsche Forschungsgemeinschaft (DFG, Germany), grant number KI1973/2-1, and the Volkswagen Foundation (Germany)—Experiment, project number 93726.

[a] Aesthetic Elite International – Private Clinic, Königsallee 88, Düsseldorf 40212, Germany; [b] Department of Plastic Surgery and Hand Surgery, University Hospital Zurich, Rämistrasse 100, Zurich 8091, Switzerland
* Corresponding author.
E-mail address: info@pallua.de

Clin Plastic Surg 47 (2020) 139–145
https://doi.org/10.1016/j.cps.2019.08.010

for autologous fat grafting, although a complete restoration in color may be difficult.

Scars that cause an intrinsic/extrinsic ectropion of the eye or lead to contractions of the mouth are regarded as contraindications for lipofilling and should be addressed by alternative surgical procedures. Moreover, immature scars are a relative contraindication for fat grafting. Scars that did not pass a maturation period of a minimum of 3 months should be treated only in special cases because, during this early period, the scar tissue undergoes a considerable remodeling processes with an inflammatory component.[2] Although the current literature does not deliver exact definitions on the precise timing of fat grafting of scar tissue, the authors do not recommend fat grafting during this period for 2 reasons: on the one hand, the true extent and character of the scar cannot be assessed, and, on the other hand, it is not fully understood whether fat grafting may fuel the inflammation during this active remodeling stage.

Patients have to be carefully advised to patiently wait for complete scar maturation and undergo close reevaluation. Also, scars that may be older than 3 months but still show signs of inflammation, such as redness, itchiness, and pain, are first treated with repetitive sessions of topical intradermal corticosteroid injections. The authors specifically use triamcinolone applied by Dermojet (Dermojet, Friedrichshafen, Germany), a needleless high-pressure injection device.[3] Another rare but strict contraindication are scars that show signs of malignancy where fat grafts seem to promote cancer growth.[4]

SURGICAL PROCEDURE
Liposuction

The procedure starts with the harvest of adipose tissue. The authors prefer the abdomen (**Fig. 1**A) as the primary donor site, but other areas, such as flanks or thighs, may be selected, depending

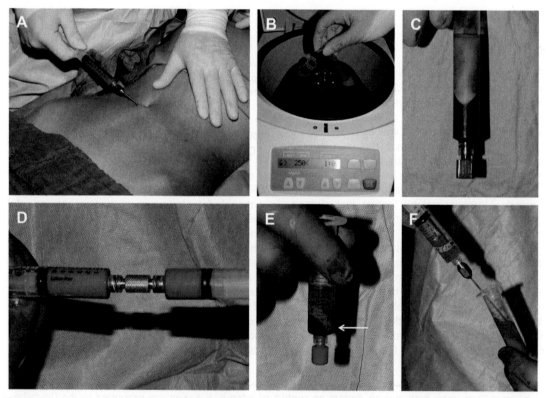

Fig. 1. Preparation of microfat and lipoconcentrate. (*A*) Adipose tissue is harvested from the abdomen, with a diameter of 2 mm, and 4 orifices, each gauge measuring 600 μm. (*B*) The lipoaspirate is centrifuged for 3 minutes at 1200 g. (*C*) After 3 distinct layers result: upper oily, central fatty, and lower watery layers. The oily and watery layers are removed; the purified fat represents microfat. (*D*) For lipoconcentrate preparation, microfat is emulsified by shifting between 3 syringes connected by a female-to-female connector for a total of 30 times followed by a second round of centrifugation (*E*) This leads to 3 layers, with the lipoconcentrate being the middle layer (*white arrow*). (*F*) The upper oily and lower watery layers are discarded manually resulting in lipoconcentrate remaining lipoconcentrate

on the preference of the performing plastic surgeon and patient.[5] The authors investigated the content of soluble factors, stromal vascular fraction (SVF) cells, and ASCs in lipoaspirates from the abdomen, knee, and thighs earlier.[5] Although the content of matrix metalloproteinase (MMP)-9 was significantly higher in lipoaspirates from the abdomen compared with the knee, the concentration of other growth factors, SVF cells, and ASC count showed no statistical difference between the 3 donor sites. Therefore, the authors conclude that the donor site for fat harvest can be well discussed with patients before surgery.

The harvest site is injected with tumescent solution containing adrenaline suspended in saline solution in a ratio of 1:200,000. Liposuction is performed by a handheld 10-mL syringe connected to a blunt-tipped thin cannula, with a diameter of 2 mm, and 4 orifices, each gauge measuring 600 μm (Thiebaud Biomedical Devices, Margencel, France). The lipoaspirate harvested by this method is called microfat. In an earlier study, the authors showed that microfat has significantly higher vascular endothelial growth factor (VEGF) and insulinlike growth factor levels compared with conventional lipoaspirates harvested by a thicker single-hole cannula with a diameter of 3 mm.[6]

Processing

For facial scar tissue, 2 different types of fat grafts generally are used: microfat and the recently described lipoconcentrate.[7]

For processing of microfat, the lipoaspirate is centrifuged at 1200 g for 3 minutes (see **Fig. 1B**). This leads to an upper oily, central fatty, and lower watery layer (see **Fig. 1C**). The oily and watery layers are removed and the purified fat is injected.

For lipoconcentrate processing, microfat is emulsified by shifting between 2 syringes connected by a female-to-female connector for a total of 30 times (see **Fig. 1D**). The second round of centrifugation, at 1200 g for 3 minutes, again leads to 3 layers, with the lipoconcentrate being the middle layer (see **Fig. 1E**). The upper oily and lower watery layers are discarded manually (see **Fig. 1F**) with great care not to disturb the lipoconcentrate. The remaining lipoconcentrate, a cellular suspension with low volume and high numbers of SVF cells, including progenitor cells, is injected.

Recipient Site Preparation and Injection

Microfat is injected subcutaneously through a 21G cannula whereas the lipoconcentrate can be injected subcutaneously and/or intradermally through a 27G cannula. Optionally, microfat or lipoconcentrate can be further enriched by platelet-rich plasma (PRP) in a ratio of lipoconcentrate 70%:PRP 30%. The authors commonly use the A PRP Kit (Regen Lab SA, Lausanne, Switzerland) for PRP isolation.

For flat scars and plaque-like plane scars, the scar tissue is first infiltrated with modified tumescent solution (adrenaline in saline solution, ratio of 1:200,000). After an interval of approximately 10 minutes, the lipoconcentrate is injected into the flat scars by mesotherapy technique (Steriject Wanted Biophymed U225 Mesotherapy Injector, TSK Laboratory Oisterwijk, Netherlands). For hyperpigmented scars, lipoconcentrate enriched with PRP is used because in the authors' experience, PRP is an easy albeit effective measure for hyperpigmentation. Similar observations were made by Cayırlı and colleagues,[8] who successfully treated melasma patients with PRP and found more than 80% of reduction in epidermal hyperpigmentation after 3 PRP sessions.

For retracted scars, the scar area is first injected by tumescent solution followed by subcision underneath the scar by a cannula. By this technique, also called rigottomy, the fibrous bands that strongly tethers the scar to deeper layers is mechanically released and then can be filled with microfat, which is subdermally injected. PRP may be added to the microfat to enhance the survival and ingrowth of the transplanted fat and increase ASC proliferation.[9] Finally, lipoconcentrate is injected via mesotherapy technique with additional supplementation of PRP in case of hyperpigmented scars.

POSTOPERATIVE CARE

The postoperative care in all cases consists of careful application of antibacterial ointment to the treated area. Administering additional heparin cream may help to resolve ecchymosis. Compression dressings, cooling, and topical/systemic corticosteroids should strictly be avoided to allow the transplanted fat grafts and PRP to exert their reparative functions and support fat grafts to settle at their recipient site. Manual lymphatic drainage should be started in the third postoperative week; gentle scar massage should commence approximately 6 weeks after surgery.

EXPECTED OUTCOME AND MANAGEMENT OF COMPLICATIONS

The whole extent of scar improvement by fat grafting with or without PRP treatment is evident a few months after surgery. During that time, the transplanted cells adjust to their new environment and gradually exert their regenerative effect. Because this is an overall slow process, patients need to be consulted accordingly. Preoperative and post-operative photographs as well as regular reevaluation may help during this stage.

Complications of microfat, lipoconcentrate, and PRP treatment are extremely rare. Minor complications include ecchymosis, pain, swelling, and light infections at the donor as well as recipient site. Major complications in the face are mostly vascular incidences that may result in skin necrosis or even blindness as reported in the literature.[10] The authors have not experienced any major complications so far by adhering to following key rules: no injection under high pressure, aspiration prior to injection, injection while withdrawing the cannula, and most importantly a detailed knowledge about the anatomy and the course of facial blood vessels. The authors also strictly refrain from injection of fat tissue into the facial muscles.

REVISION OR SUBSEQUENT PROCEDURES

In severe cases of extensive scar tissue, multiple sessions of microfat/lipoconcentrate with or without PRP may be required to reach the optimal results. Overcorrected areas may be treated by careful liposuction after a minimal interval of 6 months to 12 months.

CASE DEMONSTRATIONS
Case 1

This 27-year-old female patient presented with posttraumatic scars after injury in her childhood on the upper right lip and lateral to the lower left lip (**Fig. 2**). The vertical scar on the upper lip showed no significant change of pigmentation but a certain degree of retraction. Due to its thin straight line-like shape parallel to the rather poor developed right philtral column, the scar was fairly visible even from long distance. The scar lateral to the left lower lip showed a patch-like appearance with significant hyperpigmentation and tension that troubled the patient. Both scars were mature with no signs of inflammation. Aside from scar correction, the patient also asked for augmentation of the lips. She was informed that the hyperpigmented scar on the left lower lip may be difficult to treat in its color by a single treatment. In 1 surgical session, fat was harvested from the abdominal area. A total of 3 mL of microfat was injected into the upper lip and 3 mL to the lower lip for cosmetic augmentation, which also resulted in a better-defined philtrum as requested. The scar on the upper lip underwent rigottomy and was treated with a total of 1.5 mL of lipoconcentrate. The scar lateral to the left lower lip was infiltrated with 2 mL of lipoconcentrate supplemented by

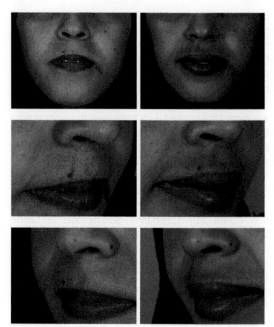

Fig. 2. A 27-year-old female patient with posttraumatic scars of the lips. (*Left column*) Preoperative frontal, right and left oblique views; (*right column*) postoperative (1 year after surgery) frontal, right, and left oblique views. The patient underwent scar correction and cosmetic lip augmentation with autologous fat. Microfat, 3 mL, was injected into the upper lip and 3 mL to the lower lip for cosmetic augmentation. The scar on the upper lip underwent rigottomy and was treated with a total of 1.5 mL of lipoconcentrate. The scar lateral to the left lower lip was infiltrated with 2 mL of lipoconcentrate supplemented by PRP.

PRP. Postoperatively, the upper lip scar was markedly less visible. The lower lip scar tissue became more flexible and less irritating during opening of the mouth and showed slight improvement in color. The hyperpigmentation was not fully improved, however, and additional surgical sessions may be performed in the future.

Case 2

This 52-year-old man patient asked for consultation regarding a facelift. The clinical examination revealed scars, however, especially on the right hemiface (**Fig. 3**). The patient had suffered a bomb attack several years prior to the consultation, where his right face was exposed to the explosion. The patient was offered a facelift combined with autologous fat grafting to treat mostly retracted scars on the right check and right perioral area. Alongside the superficial musculo-aponeurotic system (SMAS) facelift, rigottomy, and injection of 5 mL of microfat to the right cheek

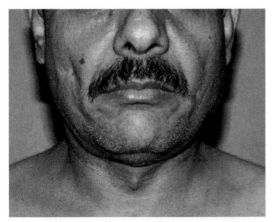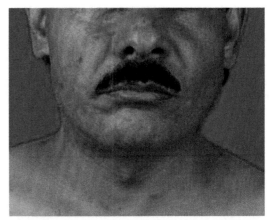

Fig. 3. A 52-year-old man with posttraumatic scars of the right cheek and right perioral area. (*Left*) Preoperative frontal view, and (*right*) postoperative (1 year after surgery) frontal view. SMAS facelift, rigottomy, and injection of 5 mL of microfat to the right cheek and 3 mL of microfat to the right periareolar area were performed.

after rigottomy and 3 mL of microfat to the right perioral area was performed. In this patient, microfat was chosen over lipoconcentrate because the retraction and loss of volume were primarily disturbing for the patient. Postoperatively, scar appearance and the overall skin texture were significantly improved.

Case 3

This 45-year-old female patient originally presented for volume expansion of her forehead (**Fig. 4**). During the consultation, several scars on the forehead were noticed, which resulted from acne in her adolescence. Although the patient was troubled by the rather small but resilient acne scars, she did not consider any further therapies as dermatologic treatment until then did not prove effective. The scars were rather atrophic and retracted. Aside from microfat for the forehead, the patient also was treated with 1 mL of

lipoconcentrate for each forehead scar. The scars and overall skin quality were markedly improved.

DISCUSSION

The unique regenerative effect of adipose tissue has revolutionized the era of surgical scar management because scar excisions and more invasive surgical measures often failed to deliver a satisfactory answer. The well-balanced combination of microfat, lipoconcentrate, and PRP injection, depending on individual indications, is the most promising in facial scar treatment, in the authors' experience. If volume expansion is aimed for, for example, in depressed facial scars, microfat is preferred. According to the microfat protocol, adipose tissue is harvested through a thin multiperforated cannula that results in smaller adipose tissue fragments in the lipoaspirate, which consequently permits the injection through thin 21G injection cannulas.[6] Thin cannulas with more liquid

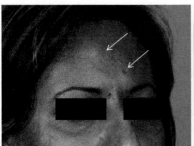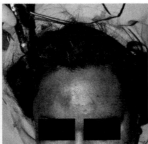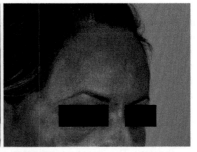

Fig. 4. A 45-year-old female patient with atrophic acne scars on the forehead (*white arrows*). (*Left*) Preoperative right oblique view; (*middle*) intraoperative frontal view during forehead augmentation; and (*right*) postoperative right oblique view (6 months after surgery). The patient underwent forehead augmentation and scar correction with autologous fat. Aside from microfat for the forehead augmentation, apprxoimately 1 mL of lipoconcentrate was used for each scar.

lipoaspirate are desirable in the treatment of the face, where even the smallest scars at the injection site or visible lumps are not appreciated by patients. In facial scar treatment, the regenerative effect of adipose tissue often clearly outweighs the volumetric aspect. Therefore, the authors prefer the use of the lipoconcentrate that condenses the lipoaspirate by a combination of centrifugation plus emulsification resulting in a progenitor-cell rich fluid of small volume.[7] The authors assume that ASCs and endothelial progenitor cells (EPCs) are mainly responsible for the regenerative effect in the lipoconcentrate. Adipocytes by contrast are disrupted through the shifting; as described previously, their intracellular content subsequently removed by the centrifugation and decantation.

The accurate molecular mechanisms of ASC action in wound repair are often debated but not entirely clear and thus need further analysis. ASCs promote neoangiogenesis, suppress myofibroblast differentiation, and modulate collagen deposition. They secrete growth factors and cytokines that alleviate inflammatory cascades and collagen production while promoting MMPs and thereby establish a higher extracellular matrix turnover.[11] Another possible mechanism is the support of keratinocyte proliferation or even the direct transdifferentiation of ASCs into keratinocytes reestablishing healthy skin.[12] Although ASCs promote the reconfiguration of the scar tissue, EPCs may foster scar remodeling by its angiogenic properties.[13] It is well known that EPCs, governed through prominent ligands, such as CXCL-12 (also called stromal cell-derived factor 1), orchestrate fundamental proangiogenic effects that make them candidate cells for vasculogenesis and wound healing.[14]

Similar to adipose tissue, mounting evidence supports the regenerative efficacy of PRP. Although PRP does not carry any cells, it delivers high concentrations of growth factors, the most important ones being platelet-derived growth factor (PDGF)-aa, PDGFbb, PDGFab, transforming growth factor beta (TGF)-β1, TGF-β2, epithelial growth factor, and VEGF as well as bioactive molecules, such as serotonine or adenosine in their granules.[15] The authors have used PRP with great success in the past few years and regard it as an easy and effective addition to fat grafting in facial scars. So far, many investigators have applied PRP most commonly as an adjunct treatment to fat grafting, laser therapy, or other regimens in scar therapy. The literature indicates a supportive effect of PRP in fat graft survival and efficacy.[8,9] The intricacy of lipoaspirate and PRP interaction, however, needs to be further unraveled to fully uncover its full hitherto untapped potential.

The authors investigated the outcome of facial scars treated with autologous microfat grafting in 35 scars of 26 patients earlier.[16] The patient and observer scar assessment scale scores significantly improved regarding pain, color, stiffness, irregularity, pigmentation, and pliability. Although no significance was reached, laser Doppler spectrometry also indicated improved microcirculation. The clinical evaluation of lipoconcentrates for scar treatment is a matter of future research.

One intractable problem is hypertrophic scar and keloid formation. Despite encouraging individual cases, the tenuous clinical data are insufficient to suggest fat grafting or stem cell therapy to ameliorate hypertrophic scars and keloids.[17] Unless firmer and more convincing results are generated, the authors refrain from fat grafting in facial scars with signs of aforementioned pathologies.

SUMMARY

In the authors' experience fat grafting is the treatment of choice for most facial scars, as either a stand-alone or an adjunct procedure. The enormous regenerative power of adipose-derived cells, first and foremost ASCs, offers incomparable opportunities in the revitalization of atrophic scar tissue. New fat graft processing methods, such as the lipoconcentrate technique, allow the intraoperative condensation of progenitor cells. Finally, fat grafting may benefit from the supplementation of PRP to unfold more of its potential.

REFERENCES

1. Pallua N, Pulsfort AK, Suschek C, et al. Content of the growth factors bFGF, IGF-1, VEGF, and PDGF-BB in freshly harvested lipoaspirate after centrifugation and incubation. Plast Reconstr Surg 2009; 123(3):826–33.

2. Son D, Harijan A. Overview of surgical scar prevention and management. J Korean Med Sci 2014; 29(6):751–7.

3. Barolet D, Benohanian A. Current trends in needle-free jet injection: an update. Clin Cosmet Investig Dermatol 2018;11:231–8.

4. Pallua N, Paul NE, Burghardt B, et al. Adipose tissue increases the proliferation of melanoma cell lines in vitro. J Craniofac Surg 2015;26(4):1403–7.

5. Grasys J, Kim BS, Pallua N, et al. Content of soluble factors and characteristics of stromal vascular fraction cells in lipoaspirates from different subcutaneous adipose tissue depots. Aesthet Surg J 2016; 36(7):831–41.

6. Alharbi Z, Opländer C, Almakadi S, et al. Conventional vs. micro-fat harvesting: how fat harvesting technique affects tissue-engineering approaches

using adipose tissue-derived stem/stromal cells. J Plast Reconstr Aesthet Surg 2013;66(9):1271–8.

7. Pallua N, Grasys J, Kim BS. Enhancement of progenitor cells by two-step centrifugation of emulsified lipoaspirates. Plast Reconstr Surg 2018;142(1): 99–109.

8. Cayırlı M, Calışkan E, Açıkgöz G, et al. Regression of melasma with platelet-rich plasma treatment. Ann Dermatol 2014;26(3):401–2.

9. Li F, Guo W, Li K, et al. Improved fat graft survival by different volume fractions of platelet-rich plasma and adipose-derived stem cells. Aesthet Surg J 2015; 35(3):319–33.

10. Goodman GJ, Roberts S, Callan P, et al. Experience and management of intravascular injection with facial fillers: results of a multinational survey of experienced injectors. Aesthetic Plast Surg 2016;40(4): 549–55.

11. Zhang Q, Liu LN, Yong Q, et al. Intralesional injection of adipose-derived stem cells reduces hypertrophic scarring in a rabbit ear model. Stem Cell Res Ther 2015;6:145.

12. Kim BS, Gaul C, Paul NE, et al. The effect of lipoaspirates on human keratinocytes. Aesthet Surg J 2016;36(8):941–51.

13. Ackermann M, Pabst AM, Houdek JP, et al. Priming with proangiogenic growth factors and endothelial progenitor cells improves revascularization in linear diabetic wounds. Int J Mol Med 2014;33(4):833–9.

14. Balaji S, King A, Crombleholme TM, et al. The role of endothelial progenitor cells in postnatal vasculogenesis: implications for therapeutic neovascularization and wound healing. Adv Wound Care (New Rochelle) 2013;2(6):283–95.

15. Alser OH, Goutos I. The evidence behind the use of platelet-rich plasma (PRP) in scar management: a literature review. Scars Burn Heal 2018;4. 2059513118808773.

16. Pallua N, Baroncini A, Alharbi Z, et al. Improvement of facial scar appearance and microcirculation by autologous lipofilling. J Plast Reconstr Aesthet Surg 2014;67(8):1033–7.

17. Lee G, Hunter-Smith DJ, Rozen WM, et al. Autologous fat grafting in keloids and hypertrophic scars: a review. Scars Burn Heal 2017;3. 2059513117700157.

Fat Grafting for Treatment of Secondary Facial Deformity

Francesco M. Egro, MBChB, MSc, MRCS, Sydney R. Coleman, MD,
J. Peter Rubin, MD*

KEYWORDS

- Fat grafting • Structural fat grafting • Lipostructure • Lipofilling • Lipoaspirate
- Autologous fat transfer • Facial grafting

KEY POINTS

- Careful facial analysis is crucial for optimal outcomes.
- Fat grafting provides a minimally invasive technique to improve facial contouring and symmetry in craniofacial patients with secondary deformities.
- The Coleman technique for harvesting, processing, and grafting provides a reliable strategy for consistent results.

INTRODUCTION

Craniofacial deformities represent a great challenge for the patient and the plastic surgeon. They occur in the setting of congenital, traumatic, or oncological etiology and may lead to psychological distress and functional impairment. Reestablishment of normal craniofacial morphology is important to allow patients to return to their normal activities and better reintegrate into society. Furthermore, improvement of the quality of injured soft tissues is important to improve the mobility of the facial region and to prevent sequelae like wound breakdown and worsening fibrosis.[1]

The transfer of autologous adipose tissue has emerged as a suitable alternative for the treatment of craniofacial deformities. Fat grafting was first described as a cosmetic facial filler in the 1980s.[2] Coleman,[3] however, was responsible for developing a fat grafting technique that allowed more reproducible and reliable results, with quoted graft retention rates as high as 90%.[4] The key steps involve the aspiration of small fat aliquots, fat centrifugation, separation of unwanted lipoaspirate components (local anesthetic, oil, blood, and other noncellular material) and injection of fat as tiny aliquots.

Fat grafting is a minimally invasive, efficacious, safe, and cost-effective technique that has low complication rates and high patient satisfaction rates. It has been used to treat deformities all over the body to improve areas with significant volume deficits. Fat grafting has traditionally been applied to aesthetic surgery[5–8] but increasing evidence is demonstrating its benefits in breast reconstruction[5] and congenital craniofacial deformities like hemifacial microsomia.[9,10] The adaptation of these techniques to craniofacial deformities from surgery or trauma seems simple but various factors come into play making its translation

Disclosure Statement: F.M. Egro and J.P. Rubin: No disclosures. S.R. Coleman: Royalties for instruments sold by Mentor, paid consultant for Mentor Worldwide LLC, paid consultant for Musculoskeletal Transplant Foundation.
Department of Plastic Surgery, University of Pittsburgh Medical Center, 3550 Terrace Street, 6B Scaife Hall, Pittsburgh, PA 15261, USA
* Corresponding author.
E-mail address: rubipj@upmc.edu

Clin Plastic Surg 47 (2020) 147–154
https://doi.org/10.1016/j.cps.2019.08.011

challenging with uncertain resorption rates. First, the facial recipient bed is now scarred and fibrotic, reducing its vascular supply and compliance to support fat engraftment. Second, the base of the zone of injury often is lined by a mesh or other avascular foreign body, which further reduces the recipient bed vascular supply and thus engraftment. A paucity in the literature exists describing the role of fat grafting to correct traumatic or surgical craniofacial deformities. Only a few small case series and cohort studies have been published, but they group congenital, traumatic, and surgical craniofacial deformities together. Nonetheless, these studies confirm that fat grafting is safe, leading to no major complications and to high patient satisfaction rates and favorable aesthetic outcomes, based on photographs.[11–13]

The authors' group recently conducted a prospective cohort study assessing the safety and efficacy of fat grafting for the treatment of posttraumatic and postsurgical craniofacial deformities. The study confirmed the safety of fat grafting with absence of major complications. Volume retention averaged 63% at 9 months, with the 3-month point strongly predicting the final result. There was no correlation between the total volume injected and retention rate. Subsequent grafting procedures had similar volume retention as the first round, leading to a significant correlation between volume retention percentage at the first round of injection to retention of subsequent injections. An improvement was noticed in satisfaction with physical appearance, social relationships, and social functioning quality of life.[14]

The authors believe, therefore, that autologous fat grafting for craniofacial deformities is a great alternative because it is less invasive and safer than traditional reconstructive options, it reaches volume stability at 3 months, and leads to positive patient-reported outcomes. This article examines the practical aspects involved in the decision making and technique of fat grafting to treat secondary facial deformities.

PREOPERATIVE EVALUATION AND SPECIAL CONSIDERATIONS

A thorough history and physical examination are the basis for successful outcomes in fat grafting. Care should be taken in understanding the deformity etiology, prior surgical treatment, and reconstructive techniques previously attempted. Evaluation of the patient's preoperative medical status must include conditions that can affect the survival of fat grafting, such as smoking and tobacco use and history of prior infection or postsurgical infection. A surgical history should be taken,

including prior surgeries, complications to anesthesia, and prior liposuction or fat grafting. A personal or family history of clotting or bleeding disorders should be noted. If there is an allergy to lidocaine, it should not be used for in the infiltration solution. A thorough medication history should be obtained to determine if the patient takes anticoagulants or supplements that affect coagulation. After a general examination, a detailed analysis of the face should be conducted focusing on basic principles of facial aesthetics, assessment of texture and quality of the skin, identification of contour deformities, volume deficiencies, scars, fibrotic tissue, and presence and/or exposure of plates or other foreign bodies. A through assessment of potential fat harvesting donor sites to determine presence of sufficient fat and assess for prior liposuction deformities to avoid worsening of those sites during harvesting.

All medications that interfere with the platelet function should be stopped 2 weeks prior to surgery. Smoking should be stopped at least 1 month prior to surgery. Throughout the preoperative planning, the surgeon should gauge goals of the patient, ensure that the expectations are realistic, and ensure that fat grafting is the appropriate treatment modality.

Indications for fat grafting include a wide range of cosmetic and reconstructive deformities. Although the procedure is well tolerated, some contraindications exist, including hematologic abnormalities and anticoagulant medication use.

SURGICAL PROCEDURE
Donor Site Selection

Fat can be harvested from anywhere in the body. Because studies have shown that the site has no impact on postprocessing fat yield, the decision of harvest site is usually based on safety, ease of access, and preference of the patient. Patients normally are placed in a supine position to provide easy access to the inner thighs, flanks, and abdomen for harvesting and the face for transfer. The donor and recipient sites are then prepared with povidone-iodine and the patient is draped in a sterile fashion.

Harvesting

Infiltration solution is placed through 2-mm incisions sites. If the surgery is performed under local anesthesia, the authors' preference is a solution composed of 0.5% lidocaine with 1:200,000 epinephrine buffered with sodium bicarbonate infused with a Lamis infiltration cannula (Mentor Worldwide, Santa Barbara, California). If the surgery is performed under intravenous sedation or general anesthesia, the authors' preference is a solution composed of 0.2% lidocaine, Ringers lactate with 1:400,000 epinephrine. The volume infiltrated is lower than the expected volume of lipoaspirate and is left in for 10 minutes. Tumescent solution is not used because of the potential for mechanical damage to fat parcels and because of prolongation of the procedure due to an excessive fluid fraction in the aspirate. Manual liposuction is performed using a 10-mL syringe and a 9-hole harvesting cannula (12- gauge or 14-gauge, 15 cm or 23 cm long, depending on the volume needed) as shown in **Fig. 1**.

Processing

The syringe is then connected to a Luer lock cap (Becton, Dickinson and Company, Franklin Lakes, New Jersey) and the plunger is removed. The syringes are then spun in a sterilized centrifuge at 1286 g for 3 minutes (**Fig. 2**). The oil in the top supernatant layer is decanted and the lower aqueous layer is allowed to be drained from the bottom of the syringe by removing the Luer lock cap. A neurosurgical cotton patty is used to wick away the remaining superior oil (**Fig. 3**). The processed fat is then transferred into 1-mL Luer lock syringes ready for injection.

Fat Transfer

The planned insertion sites for the cannulas are anesthetized with 0.5% lidocaine with 1:200,000 epinephrine before stabbing incisions with a no. 11 scalpel or an 18-gauge needle are created. The incisions can be lubricated using the decanted oil to avoid friction on the incision sites. Focal

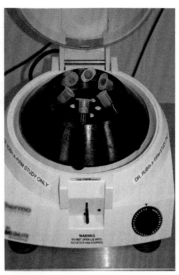

Fig. 2. Centrifugation of 10-mL syringes at 1286 g for 3 minutes.

areas of significant scar tethering can be released by subcutaneous incision using an 18-gauge needle or a Coleman V-dissector or W-dissector (sharp cannula helpful to release adhesions). A small gauge (21-gauge), short (3–7 cm), blunt cannula (Coleman type I, II, or III) is used for graft placement. The fat is infiltrated in a radial fanlike pattern at multiple tissue depths using small aliquots (0.05–0.1 mL of fat with each pass) injected as the cannula is withdrawn. The idea is to disperse the fat graft as evenly as possible throughout the deformity. Fat is injected until the desired volume is obtained or until the compliance of the recipient bed precludes additional fat transfer. The surgeon should constantly compare the treated side to the contralateral side to optimize symmetry. The surgeon should always be aware of the cannula tip to avoid iatrogenic injuries. Once the desired contour and volume are obtained, the facial incisions are sutured with interrupted 5-0 fast absorbing plain gut and the donor site incisions are sutured with buried deep-dermal 3-0 Monocryl.

POSTOPERATIVE CARE

These procedures can usually be performed as an elective outpatient procedure and can be discharged on the same day. The donor and recipient incision sites are both covered with bacitracin. The donor area is then covered with foam and postoperative compressive dressings to prevent hematoma and seroma formation. For the first 72 hours, cool compresses may be applied to the face to reduce edema, pain, and ecchymosis.

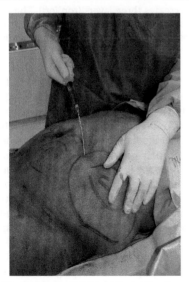

Fig. 1. Manual liposuction performed using a 10-mL syringe and a 9-hole harvesting cannula.

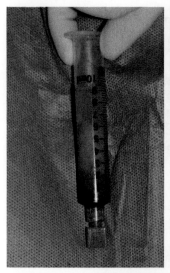
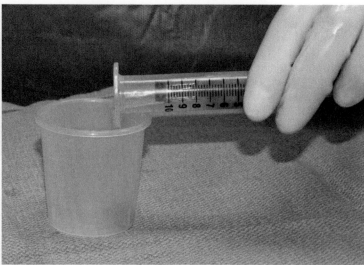
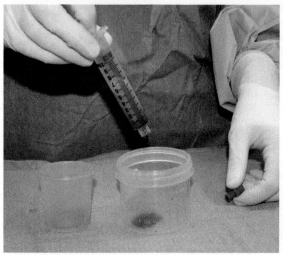
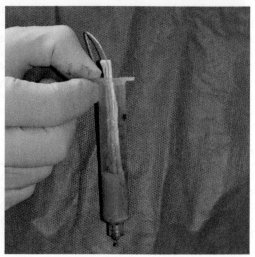

Fig. 3. Post-centrifugation processing. The centrifuged lipoaspirate creates three layers (*top left*). The oil in the top supernatant layer is decanted (*top right*) and the lower aqueous layer is allowed to be drained from the bottom of the syringe by removing the Luer lock (*bottom left*). A neurosurgical cotton patty is used to wick away the remaining superior oil (*bottom right*).

Patients are directed to avoid direct pressure, shearing forces, or deep massages of the face to avoid fat migration or necrosis.

EXPECTED OUTCOME AND MANAGEMENT OF COMPLICATIONS

Fat grafting to correct secondary craniofacial deformities is safe. All patients are expected to be discharged on the day of surgery, and significant adverse complications are very rare (none reported in the authors' clinical trial[14]). Patients can expect mild discomfort, edema, and ecchymosis for 1 week to 2 weeks. Minor complications include resorption, under-correction, overcorrection, visible irregularities, migration of injected fat, and donor site complications. Resorption should be expected to a certain degree but studies have demonstrated great variability. Irregularities or under-correction may be corrected with multiple rounds of fat grafting. Major complications are much rarer. Infections may arise from skin or mucosal flora, contaminated equipment, or inadvertent foreign body introduction under the skin. Surgeons may use Hibiclens scrub prior to the preparing the skin with povidone-iodine. Surgeons should avoid woven cotton sponges to avoid getting the cotton stuck within the lipoaspirate. A major concern with any fat grafting procedure is injury of underlying structures and iatrogenic exposure of plates and other foreign bodies. The use of blunt cannulas reduce the risk of these injuries but nonetheless care and anatomic knowledge are crucial for safety. The most feared complication is fat embolization after intravascular injection, which can lead to blindness or stroke. Surgeons can prevent this complication by using blunt cannulas (sharp and small cannulas are more likely to perforate vessels), inject small volumes to avoid a continuous column of lipoaspirate to extend all the way to the ophthalmic or internal carotid arteries, and be aware of vital structures and vessels to avoid accidental intravascular injections.

REVISION OR SUBSEQUENT PROCEDURES

Fat graft resorption rate is variable and additional procedures are often needed to achieve the desired outcome. The authors' preference is to wait at least 3 months for the inflammatory response to settle prior to the second round of fat grafting. It might be expected that a first round of fat grafting improves the vascularity and compliance of the recipient bed, which is generally scarred and noncompliant in the initial treatment. The authors' clinical trial showed that the second round of fat grafting results in a comparable retention rate as the first treatment.[14] Thus, the effect of priming the scarred recipient bed with a first round of fat grafting has limited impact on retention in future procedures.

CASE DEMONSTRATIONS
Case 1

A 31-year-old woman presented with hollowing of the left temporal region secondary to craniectomy (**Fig. 4**). Fat was harvested from her abdomen and bilateral thighs using 10-mL syringes and Coleman harvesting cannulas. The fat was processed in the standard manner using the Coleman technique, described previously. Approximately 18 mL of refined fat was grafted in the left temporal deformity. The fat was placed using Coleman cannulas (mostly with the type III cannulas). Photographs (see **Fig. 4**) show the patient preoperatively and after fat grafting (3 days, 3 months, and 9 months) with no other procedures in the interim. The patient has a lasting restoration of fullness in the left temporal region with significant decrease in hollowness over time.

Case 2

A 33-year-old man presented with hollowing of the right temporal region secondary to right craniectomy (**Fig. 5**). The patient underwent 2 rounds of fat grafting at a distance of 3 years. In both cases, the fat was harvested from his abdomen and bilateral thighs using 10-mL syringes and Coleman harvesting cannulas. The fat was processed in the standard manner using the Coleman technique, described previously. Approximately 34 mL of refined fat was grafted in the right temporal deformity during the first round and 49 mL of fat in the second round. The fat was placed using Coleman cannulas (mostly with the type III cannulas). Photographs (see **Fig. 5**) show the patient preoperatively and after 2 round of fat grafting. The patient has a lasting restoration of fullness in the right temporal region with significant decrease in hollowness over time.

Case 3

A 44-year-old man with a history of gunshot to the right face leading to ruptured right globe, loss of zygomatic arch and right supraorbital rim, and multiple comminuted maxillary and zygomatic fractures requiring open reduction internal fixation and right eye enucleation. The patient presented with hollowing of the right temporal and orbitozygomatic regions and significant indurated and indented scarring (**Fig. 6**). The scar was broken down using an 18-gauge needle. Fat was harvested from his abdomen, and bilateral thighs using 10-mL syringes and Coleman harvesting cannulas. The fat was processed in the standard manner using the Coleman technique, described previously. Approximately 23 mL of refined fat was grafted in the right upper border of the zygomatic arch, 13 mL in the right lower border of zygomatic arch, and 3 mL in the right cheek. The fat was placed using Coleman cannulas (mostly with the type III cannulas). Photographs (see **Fig. 6**) show the patient preoperatively and after fat grafting (3 days, 3 months, and 9 months) with no other procedures in the interim. The patient has a lasting improvement in the fullness in the left temporal, orbitozygomatic,and cheek regions with significant decrease in hollowness over time.

DISCUSSION

Fat grafting to correct secondary craniofacial deformities can present a great challenge because of the scarred, avascular, and noncompliant recipient bed, which can have a negative impact on graft survival. Furthermore, graft retention is also affected by the quality of adipocytes harvested and the amount of adipocyte necrosis secondary to damage during harvesting,

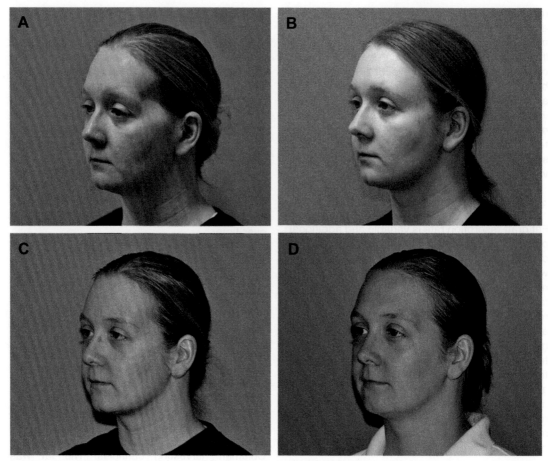

Fig. 4. A 31-year-old woman who has undergone left temporal fat grafting. (*A*) Preoperative appearance; (*B*) 3 days' postoperative appearance; (*C*) 3 months' postoperative appearance; and (*D*) 9 months' postoperative appearance. (*From* Bourne DA, Bliley J, James I, et al. Changing the paradigm of craniofacial reconstruction: a prospective clinical trial of autologous fat transfer for craniofacial deformities. Ann Sur. 2019(April 9):5; with permission.)

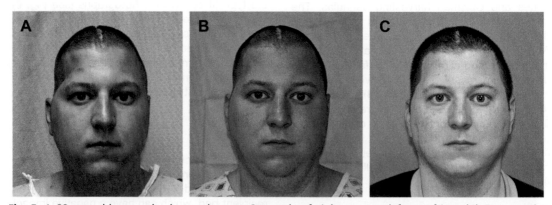

Fig. 5. A 33-year-old man who has undergone 2 rounds of right temporal fat grafting. (*A*) Preoperative appearance; (*B*) 9 months after first fat grafting procedure; and (*C*) 9 months after second fat grafting procedure. (*From* Bourne DA, Bliley J, James I, et al. Changing the paradigm of craniofacial reconstruction: a prospective clinical trial of autologous fat transfer for craniofacial deformities. Ann Sur. 2019(April 9):7; with permission.)

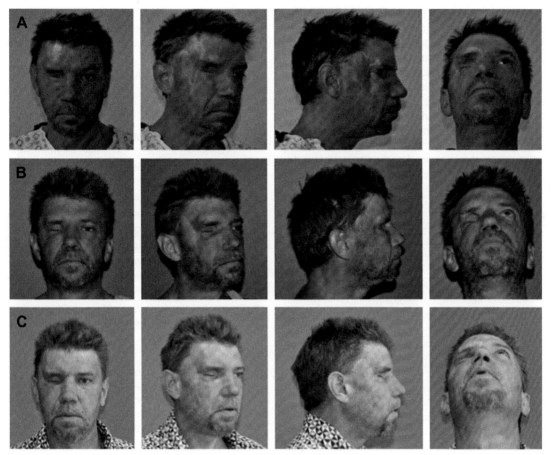

Fig. 6. A 44-year-old man who has undergone left temporal, orbitozygomatic, and cheek fat grafting. (*A*), Preoperative appearance; (*B*) 9 months' postoperative appearance; and (*C*) 2 years' postoperative appearance.

processing, and transfer. More than ever, a sound technique in the various steps of fat harvesting and grafting is needed. The Coleman technique has proved over the years to reliably improve graft retention and should be considered by the operator. It is important to avoid infiltration of large volumes, because patients with a scarred and noncompliant bed are more prone to fat necrosis, oil cysts, fat resorption, or contour irregularities. The fat should be injected evenly in a radial fanlike pattern at multiple tissue depths using small aliquots to minimize contour irregularities and improve fat survival. Fat transferred in the subdermal or intradermal layers improves skin quality, but it may lead to superficial contour irregularities and skin tears. Fat graft molding should be avoided because of the risk of fat necrosis. The surgeon should avoid danger zones and be mindful of the depth and the location of the vasculature in order to minimize the risk of accidental intravascular injection and embolization.

Although many of these secondary deformities are reconstructive cases, the surgeon should utilize key facial aesthetic principles to improve contour and symmetry. The quality and texture of skin, the amount of underlying scarring, and the level of tissue compliance should be appreciated. All these factors can impede the amount of fat that can be safely transferred, which may spur the surgeon to conduct the reconstruction in multiple stages. The authors' clinical trial demonstrated that fat grafting is safe and practical, but surgeons should be aware that a second round of fat grafting results in a comparable retention rate as the first treatment.[14] Thus, they should plan ahead and base the amount of fat transferred on the response of the first procedure.

SUMMARY

Fat grafting has revolutionized how secondary deformities are managed, moving away from invasive and complex techniques to a minimally invasive and more practical treatment option. This article has elucidated the principles used to reconstruct secondary craniofacial deformities including the fat harvesting, processing, and injection techniques. The importance of safety and optimal technique is highlighted, and evidence of expected outcomes and potential for secondary procedures is provided. A sound strategy combined with knowledge will allow surgeons to obtain optimal and reproducible outcomes for even the most challenging craniofacial deformities.

REFERENCES

1. Yaremchuk MJ. Facial skeletal reconstruction using porous polyethylene implants. Plast Reconstr Surg 2003;111(6):1818–27.
2. Billings EJ, May JW. Historical review and present status of free fat graft autotranplantation in plastic and reconstructive surgery. Plast Reconstr Surg 1989;83(2):368–81.
3. Coleman SR. The technique of periorbital lipoinfiltration. Oper Tech Plast Reconstr Surg 1994;1:20–6.
4. Parrish JN, Metzinger SE. Autogenous fat grafting and breast augmentation: a review of the literature. Aesthet Surg J 2010;30(4):549–56.
5. Delay E, Garson S, Tousson G, et al. Fat injection to the breast: technique, results, and indications based on 880 procedures over 10 years. Aesthet Surg J 2009;29(5):360–76.
6. Gutowski KA. Current applications and safety of autologous fat grafts: a report of the ASPS fat graft task force. Plast Reconstr Surg 2009;124(1):272–80.
7. Gir P, Brown SA, Oni G, et al. Fat grafting: evidence-based review on autologous fat harvesting, processing, reinjection, and storage. Plast Reconstr Surg 2012;130(1):249–58.
8. Meier JD, Glasgold RA, Glasgold MJ. Autologous fat grafting. Long-term evidence of its efficacy in midfacial rejuvenation. Arch Facial Plast Surg 2009;11(1):24–8.
9. Tanikawa DY, Aguena M, Bueno DF, et al. Fat grafts supplemented with adipose-derived stromal cells in the rehabilitation of patients with craniofacial microsomia. Plast Reconstr Surg 2013;132(1):141–52.
10. Lim AA, Fan K, Allam KA, et al. Autologous fat transplantation in the craniofacial patient: the UCLA experience. J Craniofac Surg 2012;23(4):1061–6.
11. Guijarro-Martínez R, Alba LM, Mateo MM, et al. Autologous fat transfer to the cranio-maxillofacial region: updates and controversies. J Craniomaxillofac Surg 2011;39(5):359–63.
12. Clauser LC, Tieghi R, Galiè M, et al. Structural fat grafting: facial volumetric restoration in complex reconstructive surgery. J Craniofac Surg 2011;22(5):1695–701.
13. Hammer-Hansen N, Akram J, Damsgaard TE. Clinical study the versatility of autologous fat transplantation in correction of facial deformities: a single-center experience. Plast Surg Int 2015;1–6. https://doi.org/10.1155/2015/703535.
14. Bourne DA, Bliley J, James I, et al. Changing the paradigm of craniofacial reconstruction: a prospective clinical trial of autologous fat transfer for craniofacial deformities. Ann Surg 2019;1–8. https://doi.org/10.1097/SLA.0000000000003318.

Fat Grafting for Treatment of Facial Scleroderma

Aurélie Daumas, MD, PhD[a], Jeremy Magalon, PharmD, PhD[b], Flore Delaunay, MD[c,d],
Maxime Abellan, MD[e], Cécile Philandrianos, MD, PhD[e], Florence Sabatier, PharmD, PhD[b],
Brigitte Granel, MD, PhD[a], Guy Magalon, MD[e,*]

KEYWORDS

- Systemic sclerosis • Cell therapy • Microfat injection • Nanofat • Platelet-rich plasma
- Stromal vascular fraction • Fat grafting • Adipose tissue

KEY POINTS

- Systemic sclerosis is a rare autoimmune disease characterized by skin fibrosis, microvascular damage, and organs dysfunction.
- Facial signs are frequent and include perioral skin thickening, facial atrophy, and microstomia.
- Facial manifestations are disfiguring and lead to social disability with psychological distress.
- Autologous fat tissue grafting has emerged as a treatment of localized scleroderma and patients with systemic sclerosis–related perioral thickening and mouth opening limitation.
- Cell-based strategies to enrich fat grafts is a promising option in regenerative medicine.

 Video content accompanies this article at http://www.plasticsurgery.theclinics.com.

INTRODUCTION

Systemic sclerosis (SSc) is a chronic systemic autoimmune disease characterized by progressive skin and internal organ fibrosis and microvascular abnormalities.[1] Life-threatening organ lesions only affect a minority of patients. By contrast, lesions of the hands and face are almost always present. Although not life threatening, these manifestations are obvious, hard to conceal, and lead to disability and worsening quality of life.[2–4] No antifibrotic treatment has proved effective. Unlike other autoimmune diseases, immunosuppressive drugs have a limited clinical interest.[5,6] Thus, improvement of face motion and appearance represent a real challenge for physicians and a priority for patients who often think that this aspect of their disease is neglected.

Use of adipose tissue as filling product in plastic and aesthetic surgery is an ancient technique. Significant renewal of interest in this approach was observed after the description of the Lipostructure technique by Coleman.[7] This approach, using the patient's own body fat as a natural filler to achieve structural modifications, takes advantage of its abundance and accessibility. Elective liposuction

A. Daumas and J. Magalon contributed equally to this work.

Disclosure: G. Magalon is a consultant for the Thiebaud Medical Device, and received financial grants and other support for research and honorarium as a consultant. The other authors have nothing to disclose.

[a] Internal Medicine Department, Assistance Publique Hôpitaux de Marseille (AP-HM), Aix-Marseille University, Timone Hospital 264 Rue St Pierre, 13005 Marseille, France; [b] Culture and Cell Therapy Laboratory, INSERM CBT-1409, Assistance Publique Hôpitaux de Marseille (AP-HM), Aix-Marseille University, Conception Hospital 147 Bd Baille, 13005 Marseille, France; [c] Plastic Surgery Department, Centre Hospitalier du Belvédère, 72 rue Louis Pasteur, 76130 Mont Saint Aignan, France; [d] Aix-Marseille University, Marseille, France; [e] Plastic Surgery Department, Assistance Publique Hôpitaux de Marseille (AP-HM), Aix-Marseille University, Conception Hospital 147 Bd Baille, 13005 Marseille, France

* Corresponding author.

E-mail address: secretariat.magalon@gmail.com

Clin Plastic Surg 47 (2020) 155–163
https://doi.org/10.1016/j.cps.2019.08.016

for fat transplant is nowadays considered a safe and well-tolerated procedure. Identification of the adipose tissue–derived stromal vascular fraction, which includes mesenchymal stem cell–like cells, endothelial progenitor cells, and hematopoietic cells, has revolutionized the science showing that adipose tissue is a valuable source of cells with multipotency, angiogenic, and immunomodulatory properties that facilitate tissue repair.[8–13] In SSc, the Coleman Lipostructure technique is not adapted because instruments do not enable direct fat grafting at a subdermic level or in layers that are poorly extensible or fibrotic. Microfat grafting, described by Nguyen and colleagues,[14] is now currently used to restore soft facial tissue.[15] The authors previously reported an improvement of facial handicap in 14 patients with SSc after autologous perioral microfat injection.[16] However, the clinical success of fat grafting is limited by its variable and unpredictable local survival rate. One of the most promising developments in recent years is the use of prosurvival strategies to improve maintenance of fat volume and trophicity.

Recently, plastic surgeons have added platelet-rich plasma (PRP) to injected fat, hypothesizing that growth factors produced in vivo would enhance the neovascularization, proliferation, and differentiation of adipose stem cells, improving patient outcomes.[17–19] More recently, the skin regenerative potential of nanofat grafting was studied by Tonnard and colleagues.[20] The process consists of mechanical emulsification by manually repeatedly shifting the fat between 2 connected syringes followed by filtration of the lipoaspirate to obtain a homogeneous liquid suspension, defined as nanofat, which can be directly administered to patients.[21] Because the obtained product does not meet the true dimensions required of nano sizes, the term emulsified fat is more accurate.

This article presents the authors' clinical approach using microfat and emulsified fat enriched in PRP in the treatment of the face in patients with SSc.

PREOPERATIVE EVALUATION AND SPECIAL CONSIDERATIONS

Involvement of the face, with associated oral complications, aesthetic changes, and impairment of the patient's self-image, is found in more than 90% of patients with SSc.[3] **Table 1** and **Fig. 1** show the main orofacial findings in patients with SSc.

Facial involvement is associated with disfigurement and limited expression with a masklike stiffness of the face. The loss of elasticity and the thickening of the skin in the perioral area and lips form perioral radial furrowing and narrowing of the oral aperture, leading to mouth opening reduction that interferes considerably with basic functions such as eating, speaking, oral hygiene, and professional dental care. Furthermore, xerostomia because of salivary gland fibrosis and reduced saliva production increases the risk of periodontal diseases and caries.[3,22,23]

Table 1
Orofacial findings in patients with systemic sclerosis

Orofacial Findings	Commentaries
Skin sclerosis of the face	Very frequent, around 90% of cases. The face becomes amimic, cutaneous wrinkles disappear, vertical furrows develop around the mouth caused by retraction of the skin, the nose becomes sharp and lips thin
Telangiectasia	Especially located in the face, lips, or the inside of the mouth, they can lead to severe aesthetic concerns
Skin pigmentation abnormalities	Hypopigmentation and hyperpigmentation mostly observed in the diffuse cutaneous form of scleroderma. Vitiligo is possible
Sicca syndrome	Sicca syndrome is detected in approximately 70% of patients with SSc. It is secondary to salivary gland fibrosis
Diminished mouth opening	Frequent, around 60%. Thinning of lips and reduction of mouth width (microcheilia) and opening (microstomia) with, as a consequence, difficult dental care
Osteolysis of mandibular angles	Mandibular bone resorption is mainly encountered in patients with marked facial skin fibrosis: chewing and swallowing movements may be impaired, pain is often reported
Altered dentition and difficulties during dental care	Oromucosal involvement include ulcerations, dry mouth, periodontitis, wide periodontal ligament space, dental root resorption, and loose teeth

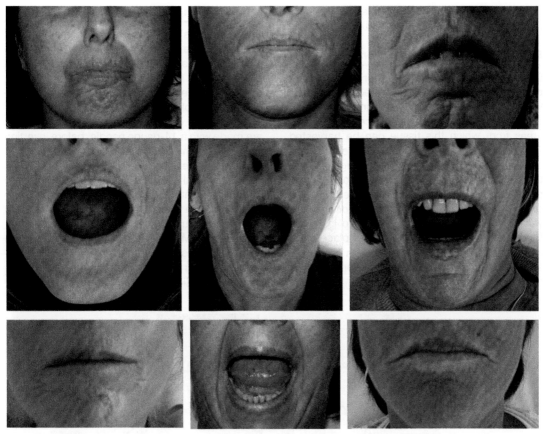

Fig. 1. Various aspects of SSc face involvement, showing skin sclerosis, cutaneous wrinkles, vertical furrows around the mouth, sharp nose and lip retraction, telangiectasia, hypopigmentation and hyperpigmentation, and reduction of mouth opening.

Several validated tools have been developed for assessment of the involvement of the face. Skin involvement is usually assessed by the Rodnan skin score. This semiquantitative score rates the severity of skin sclerosis from 0 (normal) to 3 (most severe). Xerostomia can be easily measured by sugar test (time to melt a sugar cube on the tongue, without crunching it) and with the Xerostomia Inventory Index. Mouth opening is assessed in centimeters by measuring the distance between the tips of upper and lower incisor teeth. Elastosonography and three-dimensional photographs can also be used. Mouth-related disability can be assessed by the Mouth Handicap in Systemic Sclerosis (MHISS) scale, which is the first mouth-specific disability outcome measure designed for patients with SSc.[3] This scale evaluates 3 factors: reduced mouth opening, sicca syndrome, and aesthetic concerns. The MHISS score explained up to 36% of the variance of the Heath Assessment Questionnaire score. This finding highlights the need to specifically assess disability involving the mouth in patients with SSc. Rehabilitation

and management of the face is mainly based on physiotherapy with mimic exercises, massage, and self-administered home-based exercises. Mouth care and dental care are not specific.

SURGICAL TECHNIQUE USING MICROFAT AND EMULSIFIED FAT–ENRICHED PLATELET-RICH PLASMA

Reinjection of autologous fat tissue has volumizing and trophic properties. Coleman[7] formalized the technique and nowadays most surgeons consider adipose tissue to be the ideal filler. However, the special context of SSc requires certain modifications to this approach; in particular, the use of harvest and implantation of smaller morsels or packets of adipose tissue.[14] Thus, microfat grafting has been the first evolution of the art. This minimally invasive technique is now enriched with PRP, which contains high level of growth factors to improve microfat retention. Treatment of face disability in patients with SSc is currently completed with emulsified fat enriched with PRP for regenerative purposes, which has the advantage of passing through smaller needles (25–30 gauge) (Video 1).

Patient and Donor Site Selection

During the first consultation (after a clinical and photographic analysis), the surgeon checks the venous access for blood harvesting and defines the amount of adipose tissue necessary and the areas from which this tissue can be harvested. Preferred harvesting areas include the inner side of the knees, abdomen, external thigh, internal thigh, and back. The preferred location for small quantities is the inner side of the knees. In cases of previous adipose tissue harvesting or cryolipolysis, a nontreated area is preferred to avoid any fibrosis tissue. The procedure takes place under local anesthesia (supplemented with conscious sedation if needed) and can be performed either as outpatient or inpatient care.

Infiltration and Microfat Sampling

The first step is anesthesia of the entry points with a small syringe and a 30-gauge needle with pure lidocaine 1% and epinephrine (1 mg/L) to avoid bleeding. For infiltration of the harvested area, the authors use a modified Klein solution containing 200 mL of physiologic serum and 40 mL of lidocaine 1% and epinephrine (1 mg/L). Entry points are made with a 14-gauge needle, before inserting the infiltration/harvesting St'rim cannula (Thiebaud Biomedical Devices, Paris, France; 14 gauge, 2-mm external diameter, 8 holes of 0.58 mm square). Infiltration is performed in a closed system between a bag containing anesthetic solution and a cannula using the 3-way valve Fat Lock System (Benew Medical, Melesse, France) (yellow) (**Fig. 2**D). Diffusion of the anesthetic solution during 10 minutes before microfat harvesting is recommended. Microfat is harvested with the same

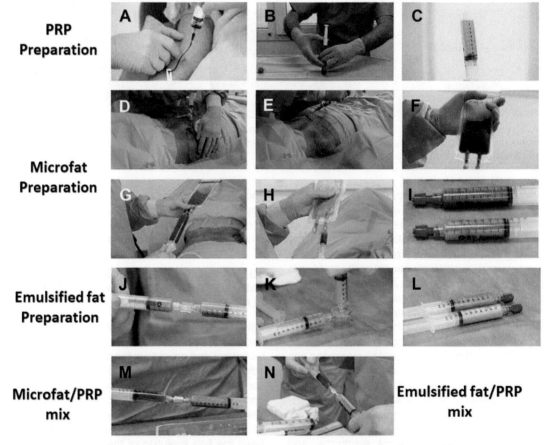

Fig. 2. Preparation of the regenerative products for facial disability treatment of patients with SSc. (*A*) Aseptic harvesting of the blood. (*B*) Preparation of PRP. (*C*) Final appearance of PRP. (*D*) Anesthetic infiltration of harvesting area. (*E*) Harvesting of microfat in closed system. (*F*) Appearance of harvested microfat before washing. (*G*) Washing of microfat. (*H*) Recovery of microfat. (*I*) Final appearance of microfat. (*J*) Emulsification of microfat (through 1.2-mm connector). (*K*) Filtration of emulsified fat. (*L*) Final appearance of microfat (*orange*) and emulsified fat (*pink*). (*M*) Mixing of microfat and PRP in 80/20 proportion. (*N*) Mixing of emulsified fat and PRP in 80/20 proportion.

St'rim cannula connected to both a 10-mL syringe and a purification Puregraft 50 (Solana Beach, CA) bag through a Fat Lock System (red) under a low vacuum keeping the plunger in contact with the fat (**Fig. 2**E). Approximatively 45 mL of microfat was collected (**Fig. 2**F).

Purification and Preparation of Microfat

Microfat is then purified twice using 1:1 rinsing with saline solution allowing for the elimination of fluid excess, lipid phase, blood cells, and fragments through filtration by the Puregraft bag membrane (**Fig. 2**G). Approximatively 17 mL of purified microfat is obtained, and 8 mL is transferred via a Luer lock connector in a 10-mL syringe (**Fig. 2**H, I).

From Microfat to Emulsified Fat

The remaining 8.6 mL of microfat is emulsified using a Tulip Nanofat device (Tulip, San Diego, CA). Microfat is emulsified between two 10-mL syringes connected with a 2.4-mm connector (30 passes) and then a 1.2-mm connector (30 passes) (**Fig. 2**J). Emulsified fat is then filtered through the device (629 μm and 394 μm) to remove extracellular matrix fibers (**Fig. 2**K), and 7.8 mL of emulsified fat is transferred to a 10-mL syringe (**Fig. 2**L).

Preparation of Platelet-Rich Plasma

After skin disinfection, a nurse collects 18 mL of blood by venipuncture using a 21-gauge needle, filling one 20-mL syringe containing 2 mL of Anticoagulant Citrate Dextrose Solution, Solution A (Fidia, Abano Terme, Italy) (**Fig. 2**A). The blood was transferred into the Hy-tissue 20 PRP device (Fidia, Abano Terme, Italy) before centrifugation at 3200 rpm for minutes using the Omnigrafter 2.0 (Fidia, Abano Terme, Italy). A 10-mL syringe is used to recover 9.1 mL of PRP through the push-out system (**Fig. 2**B, C). Then 300 μL of whole blood and autologous PRP preparation are sampled to determine platelets, leukocytes, and red blood cell concentrations according to recent guidelines.[24]

Mixed Products

Microfat is mixed with PRP in an 80/20 proportion using two 10-mL syringes connected. Mixed product has to be immediately transferred to a 1-mL syringe before injection. After microfat/PRP mix injection, the emulsified fat is mixed with PRP in the same way (**Fig. 2**M, N).

Placement

The entry points are anesthetized with pure lidocaine 1% and epinephrine (1 mg/L) using a 30-gauge needle. The skin barrier is crossed with a 21-gauge needle in the direction in which the microfat is to be introduced through the placement cannula (21-gauge, 0.8 mm, 40-mm length). In this case, microfat-PRP mixture was injected in cheekbones, nasolabial folds, and chin for a volumizing effect. Regarding the emulsified fat–PRP mixture, the placement is performed using the same procedure but with a 25-gauge needle. This mixture is injected in an area where regenerative and trophic effects are required instead of a volumizing effect. In this case, it was injected in the upper lip, lower lip, and submucosally at the level of the oral commissure. Tissue may be injected in all areas, but especially in the superficial plane, as close to the skin level as can be achieved without risk of greater irregularities than could be corrected by a gentle massage.

POSTOPERATIVE CARE

The postoperative course is extremely simple. Patients are discharged from the hospital a few hours after surgery. No dressing is required. As typically reported after liposuction, small areas of bruising at the zones of fat harvest and local pain can be observed. These symptoms are of mild to moderate intensity and spontaneously resolve in a few days. Patients should be informed about this normal process after fat harvesting and some reassurance to them may be necessary. On the face, there are no painful symptoms, the swelling is extremely small, and there is normally little bruising. The result is stable following the second postoperative month.

EXPECTED OUTCOME AND MANAGEMENT OF COMPLICATIONS

Complications of fat grafting to the face are very rare and usually do not develop if the procedure is performed by experienced surgeons. The microfat injection technique is minimally invasive. The authors have not observed any major complications, only superficial hematomas. Complications from the donor site are the same as those expected from liposuction, and depression and uneven body surface should especially be avoided. It is often preferable in very thin patients with scleroderma to collect small amounts of fatty tissue in multiple symmetric areas. Pain and swelling are minimal and there should be very little bruising. The venous access as well as the patient's body mass index must be verified before considering the intervention in order to ensure the feasibility of such therapy.

REVISIONS AND SUBSEQUENT PROCEDURES

The postoperative assessments are done at 2 months, 6 months, and 1 year. The cutaneous trophicity gradually improves and is perfectly stable at 1 year. The authors wait for the patient's request before proposing a new procedure. In our series, a new operation is sometimes performed after the second year.

CASE DEMONSTRATION

A 50-year old woman with SSc consulted for functional and cosmetic improvement of her face. SSc was diagnosed in 2009 and was characterized by skin sclerosis under her forearm (limited cutaneous form of the disease), Raynaud phenomenon, and upper digestive symptoms with typical pattern of esophagus involvement at manometry. She was taking esomeprazole and using emollient creams on her face twice a day. Her medical history did not include any other disease, alcohol, or smoking. Her physical examination revealed marked skin thickening on the face with a Rodnan skin score for the face of 2 out of 3. At entry, MHISS score was 31 out of 48 and mouth opening was 25 mm. According to the surgical procedure described earlier, 9.6 mL of microfat-PRP mixture was injected in cheekbones, nasolabial folds, and chin for a volumizing effect and 9.4 mL of emulsified fat–PRP mixture in upper lip, lower lip, and submucosally at the level of the oral commissure for regenerative and trophic effects (**Fig. 3**). No specific medication was given after the treatment except for mild analgesics. Tolerance was good and, when asked 10 days later, the patient declared herself very satisfied.

DISCUSSION

Facial handicap in patients with SSc is often overlooked, but it is highly important for the patient's quality of life, and therapeutic approaches are lacking. In recent decades, autologous adipose tissue grafting has been successfully used to treat several clinical conditions characterized by skin atrophy or fibrosis, such as radiodermatitis, burning sequelae, linear scleroderma, and morphea.

The authors were the first to show, in an open-label, monocentric trial among 14 patients with SSc, the benefits of subcutaneous perioral microfat injection in the treatment of facial handicap, skin sclerosis, mouth opening limitation, sicca syndrome, and facial pain.[16] Del Papa and colleagues[25] also reported a significant clinical improvement in oral opening in 20 patients with SSc using the Coleman method.

At present, the goal of mixing products is to enhance fat graft survival and improve skin trophicity. The goal of adding PRP to autologous fat graft is to increase the survival rate of the graft and improve the cutaneous trophicity above the grafted areas. PRP is described as having a role in increasing fat graft survival by providing nutrient support from its plasma component and enhancing the proliferation of preadipocytes through the secretion of a great variety of growth factors and cytokines. In a recent trial, Virzì and colleagues[26] showed the beneficial effects of the combined use of autologous lipoaspirate and PRP in the improvement of the buccal rhyme, skin elasticity, and vascularization of the perioral and malar areas of patients with SSc. One of the main weaknesses in the use of PRP remains the high heterogeneity from one preparation to another, which could influence clinical outcome.[27] This heterogeneity has led to contradictory results in preclinical studies that have assessed the impact of PRP on graft survival.[28,29] The microfat-PRP mixture described in our case was previously validated in 2 aspects: (1) from a rheological point of view, in which an 80/20 mixture corresponded with a soft product[30]; (2) regarding the PRP quality, the selected device furnishes a pure PRP (>90% platelets in the final product compared with red blood cells and leukocytes)[31] and the final mixture contains around 100 million platelets per milliliter of mixture. This latter point seems important in the light of the recently reported results by Willemsen and colleagues[32] in a double-blinded, placebo-controlled, randomized trial that compared the use of fat alone versus a fat-PRP mix for facial rejuvenation. PRP did not improve outcomes in terms of skin elasticity or graft volume maintenance. However, the report does not detail either the volume or the biological characteristics of the injected PRP, but the investigators suggested that high platelet levels may be counterproductive, possibly because they trigger undesirable cellular differentiation or adipose-derived stem cell differentiation toward a fibroblastlike phenotype.

One of the novelties described in this clinical case is the use of nanofat. The term nanofat was introduced by Tonnard and colleagues[20] describing a new method to prepare autologous fat in order to predominantly make use of its regenerative properties. They showed that no viable adipocytes were left after the emulsification process, but nanofat contains many adipose stem cells and stromal vascular components. Nanofat is not suitable for filling soft tissue defects. It can be applied as a superficial intradermal filler but the main clinical application of nanofat is to stimulate

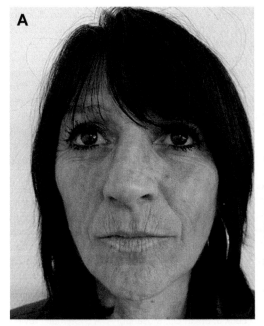

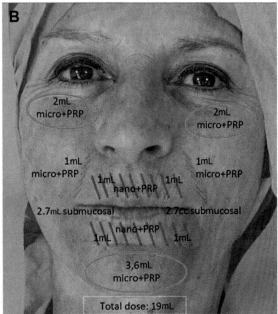

2mL
micro+PRP

2mL
micro+PRP

1mL
micro+PRP

1mL
micro+PRP

1mL
nano+PRP

1mL

2.7mL submucosal   2.7cc submucosal

nano+PRP
1mL   1mL

3,6mL
micro+PRP

Total dose: 19mL

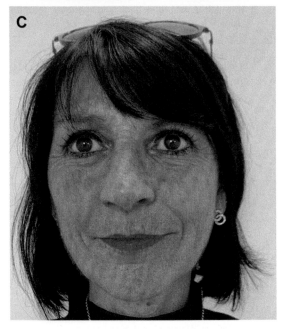

Fig. 3. Patient with SSc. (*A*) Before regenerative treatment. (*B*) Regenerative products placement and quantities. (*C*) Ten days after regenerative treatment. micro, microfat; nano, nanofat.

tissue regeneration and remodeling. This safe and feasible application makes it a valuable new tool in SSc. The authors decided to mix nanofat with the PRP based on the recent preclinical results of Lei and colleagues,[33] describing a high degree of angiogenesis and better survival with the nanofat-PRP mixture. Although the PRP-nanofat treatment in association with microfat is promising, the optimal nanofat/PRP ratio still needs to be explored.

SUMMARY

The current trend is to mix adipose cell–based therapies to improve facial disability by both volumizing and regenerative effects. Despite encouraging results and patient satisfaction, the standardization of mixture preparation and treatment methods is a pressing issue and controlled studies are needed to estimate the positive effect of PRP and nanofat or microfat.

ACKNOWLEDGMENTS

We thank all brands concerning the material used for having agreed to appear in the illustrations and to be quoted.

SUPPLEMENTARY DATA

Supplementary data related to this article can be found online at https://doi.org/10.1016/j.cps.2019.08.016.

REFERENCES

1. Servettaz A, Agard C, Tamby MC, et al. Systemic sclerosis: pathophysiology of a multifaceted disease. Presse Med 2006;35:1903–15.
2. Maddali Bongi S, Del Rosso A, Mikhaylova S, et al. Impact of hand and face disabilities on global disability and quality of life in systemic sclerosis patients. Clin Exp Rheumatol 2014;32: S15–20.
3. Mouthon L, Rannou F, Bérezné A, et al. Development and validation of a scale for mouth handicap in systemic sclerosis: the Mouth Handicap in Systemic Sclerosis scale. Ann Rheum Dis 2007;66: 1651–5.
4. Rannou F, Poiraudeau S, Berezné A, et al. Assessing disability and quality of life in systemic sclerosis: construct validities of the Cochin hand function scale, Health assessment Questionnaire (HAQ), systemic sclerosis HAQ, and medical outcomes study 36-item short form Health Survey. Arthritis Rheum 2007;57:94–102.
5. Kowal-Bielecka O, Landewé R, Avouac J, et al. EULAR recommendations for the treatment of systemic sclerosis: a report from the EULAR Scleroderma Trials and Research group (EUSTAR). Ann Rheum Dis 2009;68:620–8.
6. Pope JE, Bellamy N, Seibold JR, et al. A randomized, controlled trial of methotrexate versus placebo in early diffuse scleroderma. Arthritis Rheum 2001;44: 1351–8.
7. Coleman SR. Structural fat grafting: more than a permanent filler. Plast Reconstr Surg 2006;118: 108S–20S.
8. Gimble JM, Katz AJ, Bunnell BA. Adipose-derived stem cells for regenerative medicine. Circ Res 2007;100:1249–60.
9. Zuk PA, Zhu M, Ashjian P, et al. Human adipose tissue is a source of multipotent stem cells. Mol Biol Cell 2002;13:4279–95.
10. Kapur SK, Katz AJ. Review of the adipose derived stem cell secretome. Biochimie 2013;95:2222–8.
11. Leto Barone AA, Khalifian S, Lee WP, et al. Immunomodulatory effects of adipose-derived stem cells: fact or fiction? Biomed Res Int 2013;2013: 383685.
12. Rehman J, Traktuev D, Li J, et al. Secretion of angiogenic and antiapoptotic factors by human adipose stromal cells. Circulation 2004;109:1292–8.
13. Scuderi N, Ceccarelli S, Onesti MG, et al. Human adipose-derived stromal cells for cell-based therapies in the treatment of systemic sclerosis. Cell Transplant 2013;22:779–95.
14. Nguyen PS, Desouches C, Gay AM, et al. Development of micro-injection as an innovative autologous fat graft technique: the use of adipose tissue as dermal filler. J Plast Reconstr Aesthet Surg 2012; 65:1692–9.
15. Alharbi Z, Opländer C, Almakadi S, et al. Conventional vs. micro-fat harvesting: how fat harvesting technique affects tissue-engineering approaches using adipose tissue-derived stem/stromal cells. J Plast Reconstr Aesthet Surg 2013;66:1271–8.
16. Sautereau N, Daumas A, Truillet R, et al. Efficacy of autologous microfat graft on facial handicap in systemic sclerosis patients. Plast Reconstr Surg Glob Open 2016;4:e660.
17. Luck J, Smith OJ, Mosahebi A. A Systematic review of autologous platelet-rich plasma and fat graft preparation methods. Plast Reconstr Surg Glob Open 2017;5:e1596.
18. Serra-Mestre JM, Serra-Renom JM, Martinez L, et al. Platelet-rich plasma mixed-fat grafting: a reasonable prosurvival strategy for fat grafts ? Aesthetic Plast Surg 2014;38:1041–9.
19. Jin R, Zhang L, Zhang Y-G. Does platelet-rich plasma enhance the survival of grafted fat ? An update review. Int J Clin Exp Med 2013;6:252–8.
20. Tonnard P, Verpaele A, Peeters G, et al. Nanofat grafting: basic research and clinical applications. Plast Reconstr Surg 2013;132:1017–26.
21. Alexander RW. Understanding mechanical emulsification (Nanofat) versus enzymatic isolation of tissue stromal vascular fraction (tSVF) cells from adipose tissue: potential uses in biocellular regenerative medicine. J Prolotherapy 2016;8:e947–60.
22. Wood RE, Lee P. Analysis of the oral manifestations of systemic sclerosis (scleroderma). Oral Surg Oral Med Oral Pathol 1988;65:172–8.
23. Vincent C, Agard C, Barbarot S, et al. Orofacial manifestations of systemic sclerosis: a study of 30 consecutive patients. Rev Med Interne 2009;30:5–11.
24. Graiet H, Lokchine A, Francois P, et al. Use of platelet-rich plasma in regenerative medicine: technical tools for correct quality control. BMJ Open Sport Exerc Med 2018;4:e000442.
25. Del Papa N, Caviggioli F, Sambataro D, et al. Autologous fat grafting in the treatment of fibrotic perioral changes in patients with systemic sclerosis. Cell Transplant 2015;24:63–72.
26. Virzi F, Bianca P, Giammona A, et al. Combined platelet-rich plasma and lipofilling treatment provides great improvement in facial skin-induced lesion

regeneration for scleroderma patients. Stem Cell Res Ther 2017;8:236.

27. Magalon J, Bausset O, Serratrice N, et al. Characterization and comparison of 5 platelet-rich plasma preparations in a single-donor model. Arthroscopy 2014;30:629–38.

28. Nakamura S, Ishihara M, Takikawa M, et al. Platelet-rich plasma (PRP) promotes survival of fat-grafts in rats. Ann Plast Surg 2010;65:101–6.

29. Por Y-C, Yeow VK-L, Louri N, et al. Platelet-rich plasma has no effect on increasing free fat graft survival in the nude mouse. J Plast Reconstr Aesthet Surg 2009;62:1030–4.

30. Ghazouane R, Bertrand B, Philandrianos C, et al. What about the rheological properties of PRP/ microfat mixtures in fat grafting procedure? Aesthetic Plast Surg 2017;41:1217–21.

31. Guillibert C, Charpin C, Raffray M, et al. Single injection of high volume of autologous pure PRP provides a significant improvement in knee Osteoarthritis: a prospective routine care study. Int J Mol Sci 2019; 15:20.

32. Willemsen JCN, Van Dongen J, Spiekman M, et al. The addition of platelet-rich plasma to facial lipofilling: a double-blind, placebo-controlled, randomized trial. Plast Reconstr Surg 2018;141:331–43.

33. Lei X, Liu H, Pang M, et al. Effects of platelet-rich plasma on fat and nanofat survival: an experimental study on mice. Aesthetic Plast Surg 2019;43(4): 1085–94.

Prevention and Management of Serious Complications After Facial Fat Grafting

Ping Song, MD[a], Xiao Xu, MD[b], Minliang Chen, MD, PhD[b],
Lee L.Q. Pu, MD, PhD[c],*

KEYWORDS

- Facial fat grafting • Complications • Prevention • Management

KEY POINTS

- Facial fat grafting, in general, is considered a safe procedure with a very low complication rate.
- Incidences of complications, especially some serious ones, are possibly underreported.
- Prevention of complications relies on mastery of local anatomy and emphasis on safe techniques.
- Complication management begins with high index of suspicion, early diagnosis, and prompt treatment.

INTRODUCTION

Facial fat grafting has become a popular adjunct to facial rejuvenation, contouring, or regenerative surgery. However, as the prevalence of this procedure increases, the incidences of serious complications after facial fat grafting are also rising. This may be especially true with less experienced surgeons. As of this writing, the literature contains only on a handful of case reports. However, complications may be underreported and thus the incidence of more serious complications may be higher. Serious complications include infections and injury to important structures, such as the globe, as well as fat emboli into the brain. In this article, the authors review reported serious complications after facial fat grafting and provide their expert opinions on how those complications could potentially be prevented. Furthermore, proper management of each type of complication after facial fat grafting is outlined.

REPORTED SERIOUS COMPLICATIONS

One of the largest retrospective series, by Kim and colleagues,[1] reviewed 1261 patients who underwent full-face fat grafting for augmentation and found 62 patients (4.9%) who developed moderate complications. This included chronic swelling, fibrosis, acne, headaches, and irregularity after injection. They did not find any severe complications in their cohort.

However, there have been case reports and small case series that do highlight the severe complications that can occur following facial fat grafting. There have been no extensive reports of serious infections associated with facial fat grafting. However, the literature does contain reported cases of atypical mycobacterial infections

Disclosure Statement: The authors have nothing to disclose.
[a] Division of Plastic Surgery, University of California Medical Center, Sacramento, CA, USA; [b] Department of Plastic and Burn Surgery, The Third Medical Center of Chinese PLA General Hospital, Beijing, China; [c] Division of Plastic Surgery, University of California Davis Medical Center, 2335 Stockton Boulevard, Suite 6008, Sacramento, CA 95817, USA
* Corresponding author.
E-mail address: llpu@ucdavis.edu

following facial fat grafting.[2–4] Interestingly, a report of atypical mycobacterial infection was found following rhytidectomy and neck lift,[5] without fat grafting as an adjunct. More recently, there are reports of atypical mycobacterial infection following facial fat grafting with the use of cryopreserved autologous fat,[2,3] as well as fresh autologous fat.[4] Additionally, fat grafting was used as an adjunct to a transconjunctival lower blepharoplasty in 1 such case.[4] All cases resolved with antibiotics, with or without additional surgical interventions, but the patients were left with contour irregularities, scarring, and hyperpigmentation.

However, there are small numbers of case reports that do highlight loss of vision, as well as cerebral infarct, as a rare complication.[6–11] Early case reports by Teimourian,[6] as well as Feinendegen[7] a decade later, highlight such dreaded complications. In the former, immediate ocular pain and subsequent permanent vision loss was noted; whereas, in the latter, complications were seen 7 hours postinjection with both cerebral and retinal infarcts. The proposed mechanism is likely a combination of anatomy and technique. High pressure generated within a relatively small area can force particles of fat into the arterial arcade of the face. The pressure leads to retrograde flow within the arterial system, often from a terminal branch of the ophthalmic artery (ie, supratrochlear or dorsal nasal artery), which then can embolize to the central retinal artery or propel more centrally into the internal carotid artery. A 2012 systematic review found 15 reports of blindness following facial cosmetic fat grafting.[12] In all cases, the signs and symptoms of an adverse effect were seen almost immediately. All patients complained of ocular pain and loss of vision, and 3 patients experienced additional central nervous system deficits resulting from cerebral infarct secondary to fat emboli. Although the data are incomplete, the review does highlight certain suboptimal techniques. These include use of 10 cm^3 and 20 cm^3 syringes for injection, as well as the use of sharp needles for injection. Tragically, there has been 1 case report of a fatal stroke following facial fat injection in the neurology literature.[13]

PREVENTION OF COMPLICATIONS

The importance of prevention is paramount in avoiding serious complications following facial fat grafting. The keys to prevention are knowing the anatomy, appropriate recipient site preparation, and safe injection technique. The head and neck anatomy is arguably one of complexities and nuances. Knowing the key anatomy and landmarks is central in providing safety for the patient. There are several review articles that dive deeper into the regional anatomy of the upper, middle, and lower thirds of the face.[14–16] Specific areas of interest include the temporal region, the periorbital, and the nasal region. A 2017 cadaveric study of the temporal region highlight 4 separate fat compartments as ideal targets for fat grafting.[14] The investigators also define an anatomic danger zone of caution, which contains the sentinel vein, perforating vessels, and branches of the facial nerve (Fig. 1). From this study, the investigators

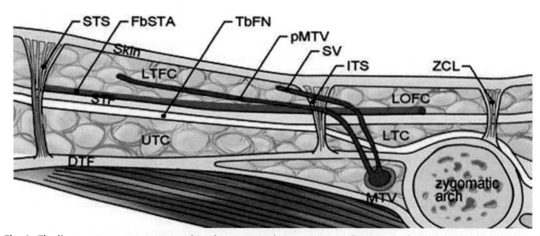

Fig. 1. The ligamentous, compartmental, and neurovascular structures in the temporal region. DTF, Deep temporal fascia; FbSTA, Frontal branch of Superficial Temporal Artery; ITS, Inferior temporal septum; LOFC, Lateral orbital fat compartment; LTC, Lower temporal compartment; LTFC, Lateral temporal-cheek fat compartment; MTV, Middle temporal vein; ORL, Orbital retaining ligament; pMTV, Perforator of MTV; STF, Superior temporal fascia; STS, Superior temporal septum; SV, Sentinel vein; pMTV, Perforator of MTV; UTC, Upper temporal compartment; ZCL, Zygomatic cutaneous ligament. (*From* Huang R-L, Xie Y, Wang W, et al. Anatomical study of temporal fat compartments and its clinical application for temporal fat grafting. Aesthet Surg J. 2017;37(8):858; with permission.)

recommend a safe site of cannula insertion, as well as a technique to address the deep and superficial fat compartments.

Specific to the periorbital and perinasal anatomy, a recent 2018 meta-analysis found 48 new cases of filler-induced vision changes in a 3-year period.[15] Only 1 case reported the use of autologous fat. The investigators found the most common location of injection that caused vision changes were in the nasal region (56%), followed by the glabella (27%), and forehead (18%). They highlight the local vascular anatomy and the importance of recognizing high-risk areas such as the glabella and perinasal region. Surgeons should be cautious of their injection plane, which is often safest on the bone or periosteum, or superficial in the dermis. Additionally, there are many variable vascular arcades in these regions that can all be put at risk for embolic events, especially if safe injection technique is not strictly adhered to. One of the most vulnerable periorbital vessels is the ophthalmic artery. It has many branches, including the supraorbital and supratrochlear arteries, as well as the dorsal nasal artery (**Fig. 2**). Each of these superficial arteries can be injured during autologous lipofilling, thus acting as a retrograde channel to the ophthalmic artery via strong retrograde pressure-induced embolization.

The perinasal vasculature also has anastomosis with the previously mentioned branches from the ophthalmic artery. The facial artery and its terminal branches, such as the angular artery, also share anastomotic arcades with the supratrochlear and infraorbital arteries. Again, the safest location for injection is deep, on the bone or cartilage, or within the dermis. However, it is tempting to inject within the subcutaneous tissue plane, especially within stronger rhytides, such as the nasolabial fold, or to augment nasal shape and projection (**Fig. 3**). However, the facial artery and its branches course within this region and thus are susceptible to cannulation or embolization, possibly accounting for why perinasal injections are responsible for most complications seen in a recent review.[15] In the worst case scenario, overfilling and the subsequent pressure gradient can lead to even more proximal embolic phenomenon within the internal carotid artery and, therefore, into the central nervous system.

The middle third of the face also important to master if safe lipofilling is to be performed. Important vascular structures, such as the facial artery and vein, as well as the angular vessels, must be avoided. Additionally, the depth of the injection is important to address the natural process of aging. There is the concept of targeted volume restoration for the midface, according to physiologic fat compartments. Specifically, the deep medial

cheek fat comprises 2 compartments, medial and latera, separated by fascia arising from the levator angulus oris muscle. Safe lipofilling can be achieved in this important deeper compartment through a perioral commissure incision, as the surgeon builds up the support under the superficial malar fat, restoring the characteristic appearance of a youthful cheek.[16] Further understanding of facial anatomy and knowledge of optimized techniques will ensure safe and efficacious delivery of results. The surgeon must always be mindful of the important neurovascular structures in the areas of lipofilling (see **Fig. 2**A). The authors encourage plastic surgeons to review the literature to become more safe and precise in facial fat grafting.[14–17] These important concepts must be studied before performing facial fat grafting.

An additional key element to preventing severe complications following facial lipofilling is proper recipient site preparation. The authors routinely inject local vasoconstrictive agents in the planned sites of fat grafting. The standard agent is 1% lidocaine with 1:200,000 epinephrine. Once infiltration is complete, firm pressure is applied to the area to minimize the distortion caused by the local infiltration to the targets to be treated. It is important to vvait an adequate time to allow for optimal vasoconstriction, thus decreasing the chances of cannulating or introducing adipocytes into the adjacent vasculature. Finally, it is important to implement good injection techniques.[18,19] Avoid the use of sharp needles (**Fig. 4**) and adhere to proper delivery of the graft with slow and low-pressure injection, and lack of blood reflow within the delivering syringe. The authors advocate injecting small (ie, 0.1 cc) amounts of graft per pass, injecting while withdrawing the cannula, avoiding certain danger areas of the face, and injecting into multiple tissue planes, including both superficial and deep compartments of the face. The safe injection technique is described by the senior author. (See Lee L.Q. Pu's article, "Fat Grafting for Facial Rejuvenation: My Preferred Approach," in this issue.)

MANAGEMENTS OF COMPLICATIONS
Atypical Mycobacterium Infection

The theoretic mechanism for *Mycobacterium* infection likely involves interplay between poor technique, leading to increased amounts of fat necrosis, and poor sterile technique or injection protocol. When patients present in a delayed fashion, often 2 to 6 weeks postoperatively, with redness, induration, and signs of infection, the surgeon must include an atypical mycobacterial infection on the differential diagnosis. Because of the shortage of symptoms related

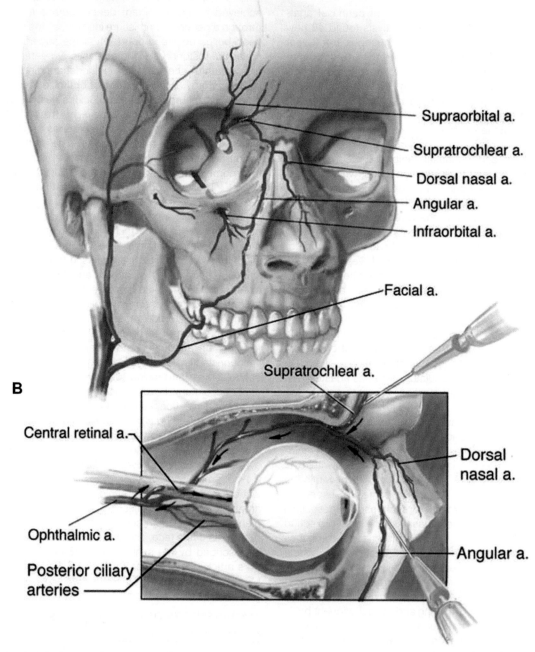

Fig. 2. (*A*) The vascular anatomy of the face. (*B*) The mechanism of fat injection inducted blindness. a, artery. (*From* Beleznay K, Carruthers JDA, Humphrey S, et al. Update on avoiding and treating blindness from fillers: a recent review of the world literature. Aesthet Surg J. 2019;39(6):670; with permission.)

to this type of infection, initial testing with routine Gram staining or cultures may miss the infection. A conscientious surgeon will always consider atypical mycobacterial infection when chronic lesions are seen or delayed redness occurs. This will allow the proper acid-fast bacilli cultures, as well as more sensitive tests such as polymerase chain reaction, to be performed in a timely fashion. The authors recommend broad coverage with dual or even triple antibiotic therapy until sensitivity testing returns. The total duration of treatment should be discussed with

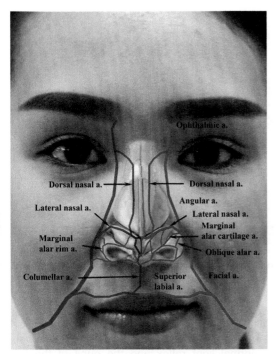

Fig. 3. The vascular anatomy of the nose and midface. *From* Tansatit T, Apinuntrum P, Phetudom T. Facing the worst risk: confronting the dorsal nasal artery, implication for non-surgical procedures of nasal augmentation. Aesth Plast Surg. 2017;41:193; with permission.

an infectious disease specialist and can often last for several months as part of an extended treatment plan (Case 1).

Tissue Necrosis

Tissue necrosis complication has been reported with use of hyaluronic acid (HA) fillers, yet is not seen in the retrospective reviews for facial fat grafting.[1,15] Yet the theoretic mechanism is the same; specifically, it results from fat embolism to terminal arterioles and perforasomes of

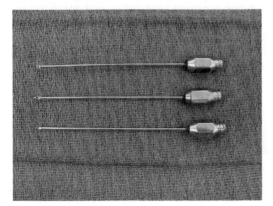

Fig. 4. Several dull tip cannulae commonly used for facial fat grafting.

the skin. There is, unfortunately, no reversal agent for fat grafting, unlike with the use of hyaluronidase for facial HA fillers. The authors recommend supportive therapy in this situation. Additionally, there may be a role for hyaluronidase in helping redistribute the fat grafts in order to decrease local tissue pressure by breaking apart the collagen matrix within the recipient site.

Vision Loss

The authors' current recommendations for suspected vision loss from fat emboli include immediate cessation if periocular pain develops because this is a herald of potential vision loss. The literature does show poor improvement in vision if initial vision loss is seen; however, treatment modalities to implement include steroids, antiplatelet agents, and possibly hyperbaric oxygen. Emphasis on early diagnosis and the administration of supportive care are critical in the early treatment phase (Case 2).

Stroke or Other Neurologic Deficits

Central nervous system complications are the most dreaded of complications. The authors emphasize the importance of early diagnosis and aggressive treatment. This depends on the surgeon having a high index of suspicion and always having a differential diagnosis if the clinical examination changes. For this embolic phenomenon, the literature reports an acute onset following injection, on the order of minutes to hours following injection. However, given the mechanism of such a complication, the key is early recognition and supportive therapy to allow for the appropriate level of care to be established.[10,12] The role of advanced computed tomography angiography or MRI can help in diagnosis and follow-up. Treatment modalities to be considered once the patient is stable include mannitol, steroids, antiplatelet agents, and possibly hyperbaric oxygen. Even though the literature shows poor long-term recovery of vision in the scarcity of severe complications, neurologic function has been reported to improve over time.

CASE DEMONSTRATIONS
Case 1

A 48-year-old Asian woman was admitted to the hospital mainly due to "infection for more than 2 months after facial fat grafting." Physical examination showed swelling of the face, forehead, and both temporal areas (**Fig. 5**A, B). The multiple previous openings were found in the

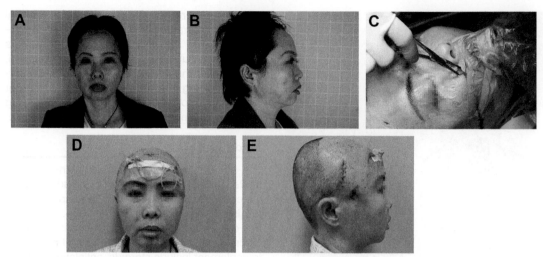

Fig. 5. Case 1. A 48-year-old Asian woman was admitted to the hospital mainly due to infection for more than 2 months after facial fat grafting.

forehead, representing incisions and drainage in the early stage of treatment at the outside hospital. An abscess associated with red and swollen skin with obvious fluctuation was seen in several areas of the face, forehead, and both temporal areas (**Fig. 5**C). With preliminary diagnosis of facial infection, she underwent multiple debridements to remove the necrotic tissue. A negative-pressure suction therapy was also performed (**Fig. 5**D, E). During the operation, secretions from the abscess were tested and nontuberculous mycobacterium infection was detected. Postoperatively, antimycobacterium tuberculosis treatment was started. In addition, local wound care, detumescence, nerve nutrients, and plasma early intervention for inhibition of scar hyperplasia and hyperpigmentation were performed.

Case 2

A 20-year-old Asian woman was admitted to the hospital due to visual impairment of right eye 20 hours after autologous fat grafting to the face. Physical examination showed no light reflex from the right eye and the pupil was 5 mm in diameter. In contrast, her left eye had a normal light reflex and the pupil of the left eye was 3 mm in diameter. The right eye could not turn up, to the right, or to the left, and the downward movement was also limited. Her left eye could move to all directions without any limitations (**Fig. 6**A–D). Head MRI showed multiple high intracranial signals on diffusion-weighted imaging and ischemic changes of the right optic nerve. With diagnosis of right eye retinal artery embolism and multiple acute intracranial infarctions, the intracranial angiography and right eye intraarterial antithrombotic therapy were performed under local anesthesia on the day of admission. Postprocedure, additional medical treatments to improve microcirculation, to reduce swelling, to nourish the nerve, to rehydrate, and to correct electrolyte disorder were also performed. On discharge, her right eye has regained light reflex and the right eye movement was significantly improved (**Fig. 7**A–D). Follow-up MRI examination revealed that intracranial infarct had been absorbed and no new infarct had been identified.

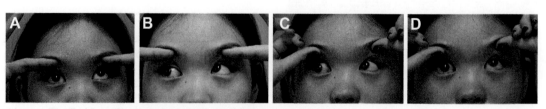

Fig. 6. Case 2 before treatment. A 20-year-old Asian woman was admitted to the hospital due to visual impairment of right eye 20 hours after autologous fat grafting to the face.

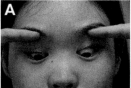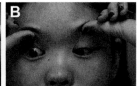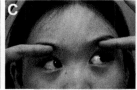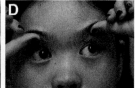

Fig. 7. Case 2 after treatment. On discharge, her right eye has regained light reflex and the right eye movement was significantly improved. Follow-up MRI examination revealed that intracranial infarct had been absorbed and no new infarct had been identified.

SUMMARY

Facial fat grafting will likely continue to grow in popularity as an adjunct to facial rejuvenation, contouring, or even for regenerative surgery. The knowledge of local anatomy and mastery of safe technique is paramount in prevention of minor or severe complications. In the management of severe complications following facial fat grafting, it is more important to avoid complications than to treat them. There have been reports of atypical mycobacterial infections after facial fat grafting. However, the dreaded complications result from embolic phenomenon to local end organs, such as the skin and eye, and the central nervous system. It is imperative to adhere to the safe and efficacious techniques previously outlined in order to minimize such complications. The authors encourage every surgeon who performs facial fat grafting to establish a systematic method to deliver safe, consistent, and long-term results for their patients.

REFERENCES

1. Kim SM, Kim YS, Hong JW, et al. An analysis of the experiences of 62 patients with moderate complications after full-face fat injection for augmentation. Plast Reconstr Surg 2012;129(6):1359–68.

2. Kim SK, Kim HJ, Hwang K. Mixed infection of an atypical *Mycobacterium* and *Aspergillus* following a cryopreserved fat graft to a face. J Craniofac Surg 2013;24(5):1676–8.

3. Kim SK, Choi JA, Kim MH, et al. Treatment of the *Mycobacterium* chelonae infection after fat injection. Arch Plast Surg 2015;42(1):68–72.

4. Chang CH, Chang YY, Lu PH. Non-tuberculous mycobacteria infection following autologous fat grafting on the face. Aesthet Surg J 2018;38(1):NP1–5.

5. Saha M, Azadian BS, Ion L, et al. *Mycobacterium chelonae* infection complicating cosmetic facial surgery. Br J Dermatol 2006;155(5):1097–8.

6. Teimourian B. Blindness following fat injections. Plast Reconstr Surg 1988;82:361.

7. Feinendegen DL, Baumgartner RW, Vuadens P, et al. Autologous fat injection for soft tissue augmentation in the face: a safe procedure? Aesthetic Plast Surg 1998;22:163–7.

8. Thaunat O, Thaler F, Loirat P, et al. Cerebral fat embolism induced by facial fat injection. Plast Reconstr Surg 2004;113:2235.

9. Park Y-H, Kim KS. Blindness after fat injections. N Engl J Med 2011;365:2220.

10. Wang DW, Yin YM, Yao YM. Internal and external carotid artery embolism following facial injection of autologous fat. Aesthet Surg J 2014;34(8):NP83–7.

11. Huo X, Liu R, Wang Y, et al. Cerebral fat embolism as complication of facial fat graft: retrospective analysis of clinical characteristics, treatment, and prognosis. World Neurosurg 2018;120:249–55.

12. Lazzeri D, Agostini T, Figus M, et al. Blindness following cosmetic injections of the face. Plast Reconstr Surg 2012;129(4):995–1012.

13. Yoon SS, Chang DI, Chung KC. Acute fatal stroke immediately following autologous fat injection into the face. Neurology 2003;61:1151.

14. Huang RL, Xie Y, Wang W, et al. Anatomical study of temporal fat compartments and its clinical application for temporal fat grafting. Aesthet Surg J 2017;37(8):855–62.

15. Beleznay K, Carruthers JDA, Humphrey S, et al. Update on avoiding and treating blindness from fillers: a recent review of the world literature. Aesthet Surg J 2019;39(6):662–74.

16. Wang W, Xie Y, Huang RL, et al. Facial contouring by targeted restoration of facial fat compartment volume: the midface. Plast Reconstr Surg 2017;139(3):563–72.

17. Mckee D, Remington K, Swift A, et al. Effective rejuvenation with hyaluronic acid fillers: current advanced concepts. Plast Reconstr Surg 2019;143(6):1277e–89e.

18. Coleman SR. Avoidance of arterial occlusion from injection of soft tissue fillers. Aesthet Surg J 2002;22:555–7.

19. Kaufman MR, Miller TA, Huang C, et al. Autologous fat transfer for facial recontouring: is there science behind the art? Plast Reconstr Surg 2007;119(7):2287–96.

Moving?

Make sure your subscription moves with you!

To notify us of your new address, find your **Clinics Account Number** (located on your mailing label above your name), and contact customer service at:

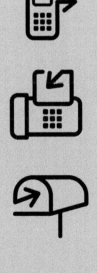

Email: journalscustomerservice-usa@elsevier.com

800-654-2452 (subscribers in the U.S. & Canada)
314-447-8871 (subscribers outside of the U.S. & Canada)

Fax number: 314-447-8029

Elsevier Health Sciences Division
Subscription Customer Service
3251 Riverport Lane
Maryland Heights, MO 63043

Printed and bound by CPI Group (UK) Ltd, Croydon, CR0 4YY

08/05/2025

01864691-0018